Instruments in Obstetrics and Gynaecology

Second Edition

Instruments in Obstetrics and Gynaecology

Second Edition

Dr. Tamkin Rabbani
M.D., D.N.B.
Department of Obstetrics & Gynaecology,
J.N. Medical College, A.M.U., Aligarh

CBSPD

CBS Publishers & Distributors Pvt Ltd

New Delhi • Bengaluru • Chennai • Kochi • Kolkata • Lucknow • Mumbai
Gujarat • Hyderabad • Jharkhand • Nagpur • Patna • Pune • Uttarakhand

Instruments in Obstetrics and Gynaecology

Second Edition

ISBN: 978-81-239-0888-5

Second Editon: 2003

Reprint: 2005, 2010, 2014, 2020, 2023, **2025**

Published by **Satish Kumar** Jain and Produced by **Varun Jain** for

CBS Publishers & Distributors Pvt Ltd

4819/XI Prahlad Street, 24 Ansari Road, Daryaganj, New Delhi 110 002, India.

Ph: 011-23289259, 23266861, 23266867
Fax: 011-23243014
Website: www.cbspd.com
e-mail: delhi@cbspd.com; cbspubs@airtelmail.in.

Corporate Office: 204 FIE, Industrial Area, Patparganj, Delhi 110 092, India
Ph: 011-4934 4934
Fax: 011-4934 4935
e-mail: publishing@cbspd.com; publicity@cbspd.com

Branches

- **Bengaluru:** Seema House 2975, 17th Cross, KR Road, Banasankari 2nd Stage, Bengaluru 560 070, Karnataka, India
  Ph: +91-80-26771678/79 Fax: +91-80-26771680 e-mail: bangalore@cbspd.com
- **Chennai:** 18/8B, Subbaraya Street, Shenoy Nagar, Chennai 600 030, Tamil Nadu, India
  Ph: +91-044-42032115, 044-26681266 e-mail: chennai@cbspd.com
- **Kochi:** 42/1325, 1326, Power House Road, Opp KSEB, Power House, Ernakulum Kochi 682 018, Kerala, India
  Ph: +91-484-4059061-65,67 Fax: +91-484-4059065 e-mail: kochi@cbspd.com
- **Kolkata:** 147, Hind Ceramics Compound, 1st Floor, Nilgunj Road, Belghoria, Kolkata-700056, West Bengal, India
  Ph: +033-25633055, 033-25633056 e-mail: kolkata@cbspd.com
- **Lucknow:** Basement, Khushnuma Complex, 7 Meerabai Marg (Behind Jawahar Bhawan), Lucknow-226001, UP, India
  Ph: +0522-4000032 e-mail: tiwari.lucknow@cbspd.com
- **Mumbai:** PWD Shed, Gala no 25/26, Ramchandra Bhatt Marg, Next to JJ Hospital Gate no. 2, Opp. Union Bank of India, Noorbaug, Mumbai-400009, Maharashtra, India
  Ph: 022-66661880/89 e-mail: mumbai@cbspd.com

Representatives

- Gujarat 0-9879558667
- Hyderabad 0-9885175004
- Jharkhand 0-9811541605
- Nagpur 0-8692091830
- Patna 0-9334159340
- Pune 0-9664372571
- Uttarakhand 0-9716462459

Printed at Mudrak, Noida, UP, India

Preface

The present book has been written with the aim of benefiting not only the undergraduate students but those preparing for their post-graduate degree as well. The book has tried to describe every instrument in detail accompanied by clear diagrams.

I would like to take this opportunity to thank my most esteemed teacher and guide Prof. K. Saxena for her constant encouragement in academic pursuits throughout my association with her.

I also thank my teachers specially Prof. S. Mohsin, Prof. K. Tewari and Prof. Z. Arshad for teaching me all that I know today.

I would like to thank my parents Prof. Maqbool H. Khan and Mrs. Afsar Maqbool for all they have done for me. I am most indebted to my husband Dr. M.U. Rabbani for his constant support and inspiration in all spheres of life. My children Shamayal and Pareesa, I hope will be able to understand in later years why I was unable to give them their due when they most needed it.

Lastly, I would like to thank Mr. Zahid Jamal and Mr. Hamid Raza who helped me with the illustrations and typing respectively.

Tamkin Rabbani

Preface

The present book has been written with the aim of benefiting not only undergraduate students but those preparing for their post graduate degrees as well. The book has tried to describe every instrument in detail accompanied by clear diagrams.

I would like to take this opportunity to thank my most esteemed teacher and guide Prof. K. Saxena for her constant encouragement and academic nurturing throughout my association with her.

I also thank my teachers specially Prof. M. Mohsin, Prof. K. Tewari and Prof. Z. Arshad for teaching me all that I know today.

I would like to thank my parents Prof. Iqbal Ali Khan and Mrs. Afsar Jahan for all they have done for me. I am most indebted to my husband Dr. M. Rabbani for his constant support and inspiration in all spheres of life. My children Shagufta and Farheen, I hope will be able to understand in later years why I was unable to give them their due when they most needed it.

Lastly, I would like to thank Mr. Zahid Jamil and Mr. Shamim Raza who helped me with the illustrations and typing respectively.

Tanjkin Rabbani

Contents

Contents

Chapter I

Instruments used for the Examination of a Gynaecological and Obstetric Patient

SIM'S BIVALVED VAGINAL SPECULUM

It is a vaginal speculum used in all vaginal examinations and operations to retract the anterior, posterior or lateral vaginal walls. The instrument itself comes in different sizes and the two blades in each instrument are of two different sizes. The blades are at an angle to the shaft and point towards the same side. They are grooved which helps in drainage of secretions by slightly tilting the instrument and can also be used for collection of specimens from vagina.

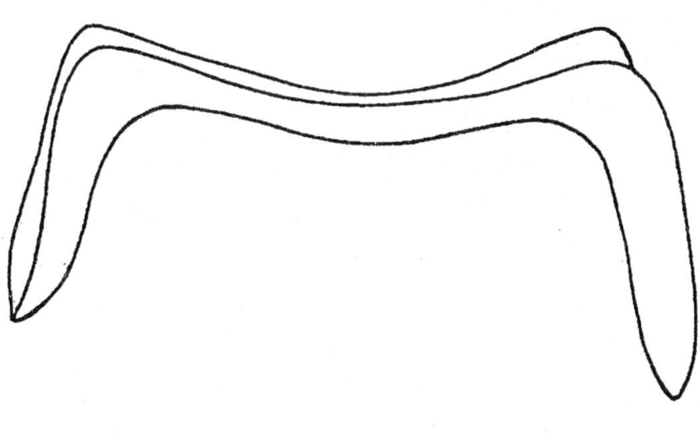

Figure 1.1 : Sim's bivalved vaginal speculum

Technique

The patient is put in the lithotomy position by the edge of the table and appropriate size of the speculum is introduced depending on the laxity of the perineum. The instrument is introduced in an antero-posterior direction. The introitus being an antero-posterior slit, this causes least discomfort to the patient and she remains cooperative. The blade is then rotated by 90°. Only 2/3rd of the blade should go in to have maximum exposure.

Uses

It is used for retracting the vaginal walls in :

I. All gynaecological and obstetric examinations known as per speculum examinations.

II. Operations on the perineum.

1. 3rd degree perineal tear.
2. Drainage of Bartholin's abcess or cyst.
3. Vulvectomy.

III. Operations on the vagina

1. Vaginal examination in APH and PPH.
2. Vaginal hysterectomy.
3. Fothergill's repair.
4. Anterior colporrhaphy.
5. Posterior colpoperineorrhaphy.
6. VVF repair and collection of urine for culture in VVF cases.
7. Culdocentesis.
8. Colpotomy.
9. Vaginal cytology.

IV. Operations on the cervix

1. Stitching of cervical tears

2. Cervical biopsies and cytology.
3. Conisation of cervix.
4. Application of Mac Donald's stitches and Shirodhkar's operation for cervical incompetence.
5. Dilatation of cervix.
6. Cerviprime gel insertion.
7. Polypectomy.

V. Operations on the Uterus

1. Dilatation and curettage.
2. Medical termination of pregnancy.
3. Endometrial biopsy.
4. Hysterosalpingography and tubal insufflation tests.
5. IUCD insertion, follow up and removal.
6. Removal of polyps.
7. Insertion of radium needles.
8. Packing for PPH.
9. Hysteroscopy.

Advantages

Gives a better field of view than self retaining speculums.

Disadvantage

An assistant is needed by the surgeon to hold the speculum during the operation.

CUSCO'S BIVALVED SELF-RETAINING SPECULUM

It is a self retaining vaginal speculum consisting of two blades shaped like the beak of a duck which are hinged together. The blades can be opened up and fixed at the required angle by an arrangement which is adjustable.

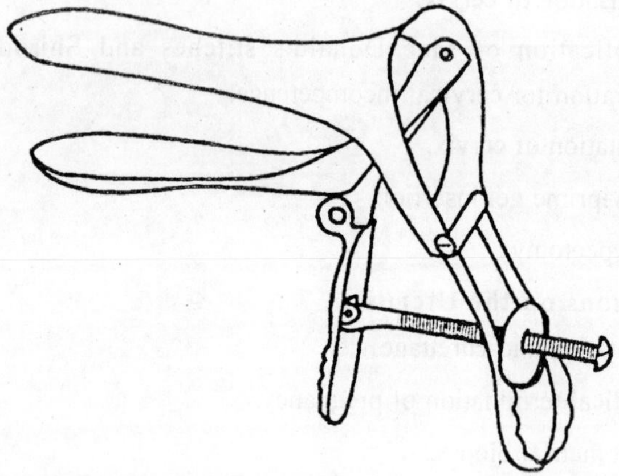

Figure 1.2 : Cusco's bivalved self-retaining speculum

Technique

The blades are closed and then introduced in an antero-posterior direction and rotated by 90° as in case of Sim's speculum to cause minimal discomfort to the patient. The fixation screw is tightened depending on amount of exposure needed.

Uses

It can be used in operations not requiring excessive retraction of vaginal walls and is ideal for operations on the cervix.

1. Cervical biopsy.
2. Pap's smear.
3. Cautery and cryosurgery of cervical lesions.
4. IUCD insertions, removal and follow up.
5. Colposcopy.
6. Used in destructive operations by Heidler's wire saw for decapitation.

Advantages

1. No assistant is required by surgeon.
2. Gives a very good view of the cervix.
3. Causes lesser discomfort to the patient.
4. Can be used in patients who cannot be positioned by the edge of the table.

Disadvantage

Only a limited field of vision is available.

AUVARD'S VAGINAL SPECULUM

It is heavy instrument used to retract the posterior vaginal wall. It consists of a curved blade at one end and a heavy lead weight at the other end and hence acts as a self retaining speculum with the advantages of both the Sim's speculum and the Cusco's speculum.

Technique

Similar to Sim's speculum.

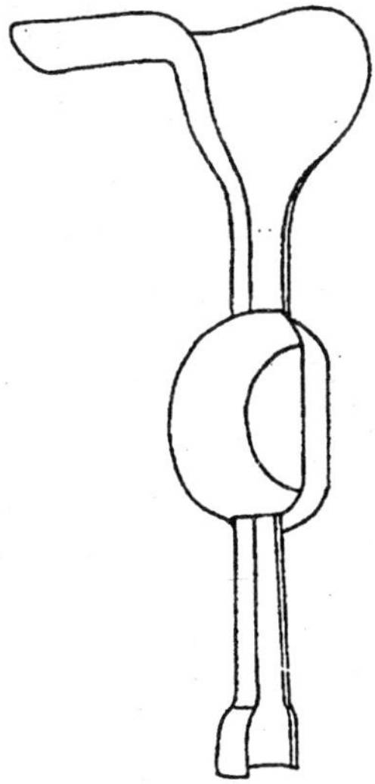

Figure 1.3 : Auvard's vaginal speculum

Uses

All operations on the vagina, cervix and uterus .

Disadvantage

As it is heavy it is cumbersome to use.

FERGUSSON'S SELF-RETAINING SPECULUM

It is a tubular instrument with no blades. It is self retaining with everted edges at one end of the tubular structure.

Technique

It is inserted gently into the introitus keeping the everted edges outside the introitus.

Uses

1. Ideal for operations on the cervix, e.g. cervical biopsy, cervical cytology, cervical cautery, Schiller's test.
2. It can be used to protect the vaginal walls during decapitation operation with Gigli's saw wire.

Figure 1.4 : Fergusson's self-retaining speculum

Advantage

No assistant is required during the operations and it provides maximum protection to the vaginal walls.

Disadvantage

Gives a limited field of vision and hence good only for cervical operations.

SIM'S ANTERIOR VAGINAL WALL RETRACTOR

It is a long instrument with a shaft and two oval fenestrated ends. The oval ends have transverse serrations and are at an angle of 15° to the shaft, and face opposite directions, the transverse serrations prevent slipping of the instrument and the fenestrations make the instrument lighter

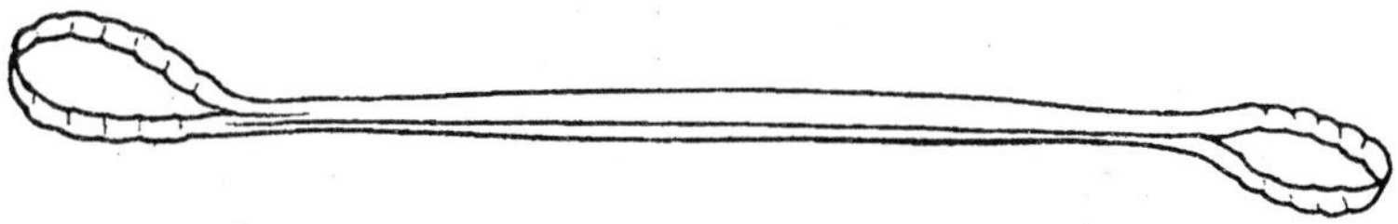

Figure 1.5 : Sim's anterior vaginal wall retractor

Technique

It is introduced into the vagina after the posterior vaginal wall has been retracted away by a Sim's speculum.

It helps in retracting the anterior vaginal wall.

Uses

1. In all gynaecological and obstetric operations requiring visualisation of the cervix and anterior vaginal fornix.
2. It can be used as a blunt curette in cases of post partum hemorrhage just after delivery when the cervix is wide open as it can remove retained products of conception by curetting large areas with each stroke.

TEALE'S VOLSELLUM

It is a long instrument consisting of 2 blades which are toothed, a joint, shank, handles and a lock. The blades are curved from the side and there is distance in between the blades which prevents crushing of the tissue held in between. The teeth provide a firm grip and the curve helps by not blocking the field of vision and causing lesser discomfort to the patient. The instrument helps in steadying the cervix and in straightening the utero-cervical angle by pulling on the cervix. This decreases the chances of perforation of the uterus.

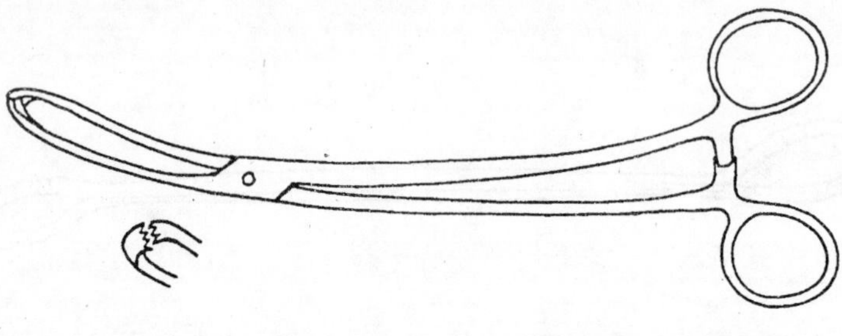

Figure 1.6 : Teale's volsellum

Technique

The cervix is visualised after retracting the posterior vaginal wall with a Sim's speculum and anterior vaginal wall with anterior vaginal wall retractor. The anterior lip of the cervix is then grasped with the teeth and the instrument is locked after obtaining a firm grip of the cervix.

The curve should face upwards so that the instrument does not abut against the lower border of symphysis pubis.

Uses

I. To hold the anterior lip of the cervix in:

1. All operations on the cervix e.g.
   (a) Cervical biopsy
   (b) Trachelorrhaphy
   (c) Cervical cautery, cryosurgery
   (d) Laminaria tent insertion
2. All operations on the uterine cavity, e.g.
   (a) MTP
   (b) Endometrial biopsy
   (c) Dilatation and curettage
   (d) Insertion of IUCD and its removal
   (e) Polypectomy
   (f) Radiotherapy: radium needle insertion
   (g) Hydrotubation, hysterosalpingography, tubal insufflation test.
   (h) Drainage of haematometra or pyometra
3. Assessment of a patient of prolapse for the degree and type of prolapse.
4. Vaginal hysterectomy.
5. Anterior colporrhaphy in Fothergill's repair.

II. To hold the posterior lip of the cervix

1. When anterior lip is diseased or friable or has a growth.
2. Culdocentesis
3. Culdoscopy
3. Colpotomy
4. In assessing a patient of prolapse to rule out the presence of an enterocele
5. Vaginal hysterectomy
6. Fothergill's repair, and posterior colpoperineorrhaphy

III. It can be used to apply gentle traction on fetal head after craniotomy for its vaginal extraction or for extracting a collapsed head of an old IUD baby.

Disadvantage

It can sometimes cause damage to the cervix when it is soft and friable as it is a toothed instrument.

JARCHO'S TENACULUM

It is a long instrument used in place of volsellum. The difference here is that it is straight and not curved and here only a single tooth is present. The blades have some distance in between and thus prevent crushing of tissue held in between.

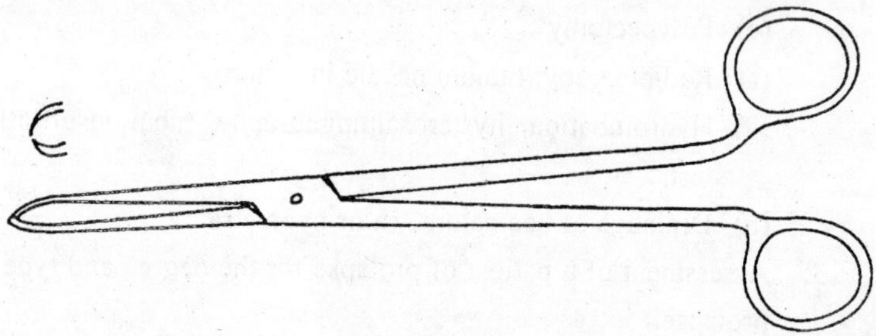

Figure 1.7 : Jarcho's tenaculum

Technique

The anterior lip of the cervix is held with the tenaculum after retracting the anterior and posterior vaginal walls as in case of a volsellum.

Uses

1. It is used to hold the anterior or posterior lip of the cervix in all indications similar to that of volsellum when patient is nulliparous.
2. It has special use in cases of tubal insufflation tests, hysterosalpingography where it prevents back leakage of gas.
3. For holding the stump of an amputated cervix.

Advantage

It is less traumatic than a volsellum as only a single tooth is present and can grip even a small amputated cervix firmly by its tooth.

SIMPSON'S UTERINE SOUND

It is a long, slender instrument about 12 inches in length. It has an angled distal end, a shaft and a handle. The angle is about 2.5 inches from the tip and is of 150°. The tip is blunt so that it does not cause injuries when introduced inside. The whole instrument is graduated in inches from the tip. The angled tip prevents uterine perforation and fits well into an anteverted or retroverted uterus.

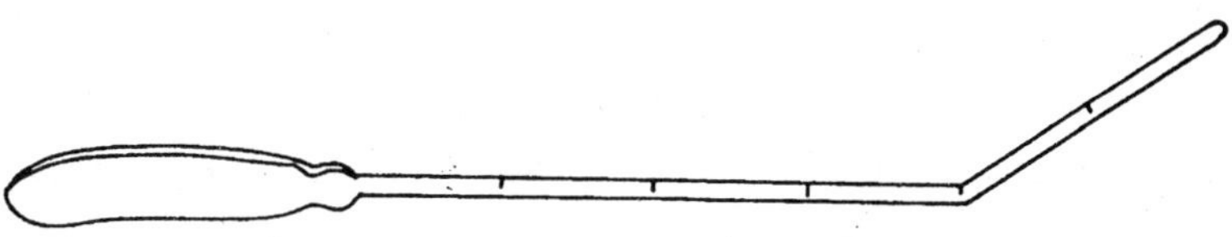

Figure 1.8 : Simpson's uterine sound

Technique

After doing a P/V examination the approximate size and direction of the uterus is ascertained. Next the posterior vaginal wall and anterior vaginal walls are retracted away and the cervix is steadied with a volsellum. The sound is introduced in a pen holding manner keeping the angle anteriorly or posteriorly depending on whether the uterus is anteverted or retroverted.

Uses

1. Measuring uterocervical length
2. To confirm the direction of the uterus, i.e. whether it is anteverted or retroverted.

3. Measuring the length of cervical canal and to diagnose supravaginal elongation of cervix in cases of prolapse.
4. Prior to most operations on the uterus and cervix, e.g. D & C, S & E, etc.
5. To diagnose any space occupying lesion in uterus, e.g. polyp, fibroid.
6. Sounding of uterus in case of missing IUCD and prior to IUCD insertion.
7. To diagnose and confirm congenital malformations of cervix and uterus.
8. To differentiate between inversion of uterus and polyp.

Disadvantage

It can cause perforation of uterus if the direction of the uterus or its size is misjudged and the sound is introduced in the wrong direction.

DITTEL'S BLADDER SOUND

It is a long slender instrument similar to the uterine sound but the differences are as follows:

(a) The instrument is slightly shorter in length.
(b) The tip is more blunt and atraumatic.
(c) It is not graduated.
(d) The angle is at a lesser distance from the tip.
(e) It is available in various sizes.

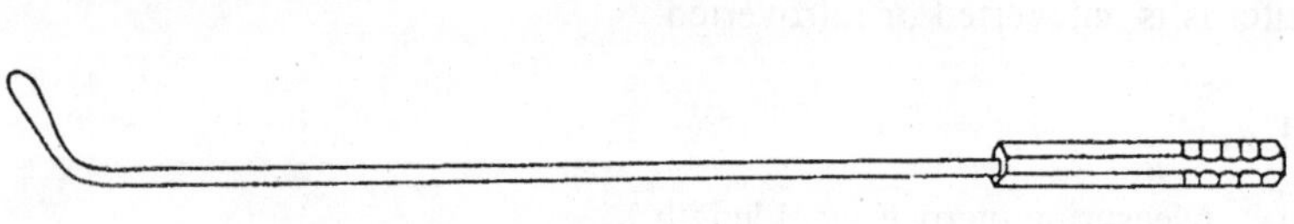

Figure 1.9 : Dittel's bladder sound

Technique

The size chosen is according to laxity of urethra. It is available in different sizes according to the English scale. A size of No. 1 is equal to 1.5 mm in diameter and the diameter increases by .5 mm for each subsequent number. 1% lignocaine jelly is applied to the urethra and after 5 minutes the sound is passed into the urethra. It is held vertically straight with the curve towards the patient as it goes into the urethra. The handle is then depressed so that it enters the urinary bladder.

Uses

1. To define the limits of the bladder in vaginal operations.
2. Diagnosis of bladder injury in gynaecological operations.
3. Diagnosis of bladder diverticulum.
4. To test the mobility of urethra in urinary stress incontinence
5. For urethral dilatation in cases of urethral stenosis. Increasing sizes are used serially in this condition.
6. To sound the bladder in following cases :
   (a) Suspicion of foreign body in bladder.
   (b) Stone

AYRE'S SPATULA

The instrument is made up of wood, plastic or steel. It consists of a shaft and one flattened blade on each end. One blade is broad and rectangular while the other blade is bifid with one tongue smaller than the other. The broader rectangular end is used to take smears from the lateral vaginal wall and the bifid end is used to take smears from the cervix and the endocervical canal.

Uses

1. Cervical cytology

2. Posterior vaginal wall cytology
3. Hormonal cytology

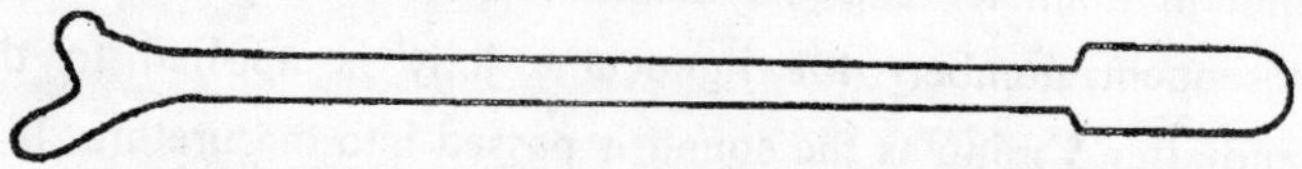

Figure 1.10 : Ayre's spatula

(1) Cervical Cytology

Cervical cancer is the commonest malignancy of the female genital tract in our country affecting women of reproductive and perimenopausal age group. Since the cervical epithelium is constantly being shed and replaced the exfoliated cells are easily accessible for screening.

A Pap's smear (1943) from the cervix can help in detecting 4–10 abnormal smears (mostly CIN) per 1000 women screened. The accuracy is about 90–95% for preinvasive grade II and III smears and almost 100% for grade IV and V smears. The false negative rate is only 10% and it is further reduced if repeated smears are taken. The procedure is simple and inexpensive with a high cost benefit ratio. Thus, it is a valuable method for mass screening of the population so that an early diagnosis is made and treatment is instituted to reduce the morbidity and mortality from this lethal disease by downstaging the disease.

Protocol for screening

1. Screening should be started as soon as the patient becomes sexually active, i.e. around 18 years of age or after marriage.
2. The frequency of screening should be at least once every year and if three consecutive smears are normal then the screening should be once in 3 years till 35 years.

3. Patients beyond 35 years should undergo yearly screening till 55 years.
4. After 60 years the frequency can be decreased if 3 consecutive smears are negative

Technique

(1) Cervical Cytology

The patient is put in the lithotomy position and the vulva is cleaned only with plain water without any antiseptic solution. Intercourse and vaginal douching should not have occurred in the preceeding 24 hours. The vaginal walls are retarcted away and cervix is visualised. The smear is taken from the cervix such that the longer tongue goes into the endocervical canal and the smaller part scrapes the ecto cervix. The spatula is rotated by 360° and spread over a numbered slide. The number of the slide is noted down for future reference against the patient's particulars. The slide is then fixed by dipping in 95% alcohol solution in a bottle within 20 sec. The other fixatives which can be used are equal amounts of ether and 50% alcohol, cytofix, hair spray, etc. The slide is stained by the Pap's method after removing it from the fixative within 24 hours. If delayed there are chances of cells undergoing changes in their morphology and false results will be obtained. The Papanicolaou's method of staining uses haematoxylin to stain the nuclei while orange G and a mixture of Bismarch brown, eosin yellow and light green, etc. are used for the cytoplasm. Last but not the least all slides should be properly numbered. Their number should be carefully noted along with the patient's particulars regarding age, parity, clinical finding, treatment received, etc. in the accompanying cytology form. This is essential for proper interpretation of results by the cytologist. The smears obtained are graded as follows :

Grade I : Normal with no evidence of malignant or atypical cells seen.

Grade II : Inflammatory with atypical cells resulting from inflammation or erosions but there is no evidence of malignancy.

Grade III : Suspicious with features suggestive of a precancerous lesion, e.g. showing dysplasia. These require colposcopy and biopsy along with treatment. Regular follow up should be carried out.

Grade IV : Carcinoma in situ with a few abnormal cells.

Grade V : Cells showing features of overt malignancy.

Grade IV and V patients should be subjected to colpomicroscopy, biopsy and curettage, etc. until the source of the cells is detected and the diagnosis is confirmed to start proper management.

(2) Posterior vaginal wall cytology

The exfoliated cells from the uterus, endocervical canal and the cervix along with secretions collect in the posterior vaginal fornix due to its anatomical disposition. The broad end of the Ayre's spatula is used for making the smear from the posterior vaginal pool in cases of suspected endometrial carcinoma. The accuracy of diagnosing carcinoma endometrium is about 70% but if combined with endometrial aspirate it is about 90% with no false positives.

(3) Hormonal Cytology

Hormonal cytology is a useful, low cost method of assessing the hormonal status of a person specially at centres lacking sophisticated hormonal assay facilities. The smear is made from the upper 1/3rd of the lateral vaginal wall as this area is most sensitive to hormonal influences. The smear is taken by the broad end of the Ayre's spatula in the same manner as for cervix and is similarly fixed. The stain used is Shorr's stain but Pap's stain can also be used.

The normal cytology consists of a parabasal layer of cuboidal cells, an intermediate layer of prickle cells and a superficial layer of cornified cells. The relationship of these cells with one another and their individual state of maturation is evaluated. The former includes their sticking behaviour, i.e. their tendency for clumping together versus a tendency to remain separate as individual cells. Also their tendency to remain flat versus a tendency for crinkling and retraction of the outer margins of the cytoplasm with a characteristic folding on itself in a navicular fashion is studied. The stage of maturation is determined by the thickness and color of cytoplasm and the type of nucleus whether vesicular or pyknotic. Dysplastic cells are not included in the study. It must be remembered that for proper assessment and correlation of findings the patients age, date of last menstrual period, parity, obstetric history and any hormonal treatment if taken should be available in the accompanying form.

Interpretation

(a) Estrogenic effect : Estrogen creates a picture of proliferation and cornification of squamous epithelium. Here the mature epithelial cells are seen as having a large size with eosinophilic cytoplasm and small pyknotic nuclei. The background is clear containing bacteria and leucocytes. This picture is known as 'cornification' of squamous epithelium.

The number of mature eosinophilic cells with pyknotic nuclei per 100 cells counted is known as the Karyopyknotic Index or KPI. The KPI is high after menstruation and falls after ovulation. It is low in pregnancy due to increased progesterone level.

(b) Progesterone effect : The pattern is predominantly basophilic with intermediate cells having large vesicular nuclei. The border shows curling of margins which is called the 'envelope effect' and the cells tend to form clusters. The picture is known as 'mucification' of squamous epithelium.

PINARD'S STETHOSCOPE

It is an instrument designed to hear the fetal heart sounds. It can distinguish between uterine souffle and fetal heart sound when the maternal pulse is counted at the same time. The instrument is simple in design consisting of a hollow tube with one wide end and another narrow end. The narrow end has a wide rim which is used as an ear piece.

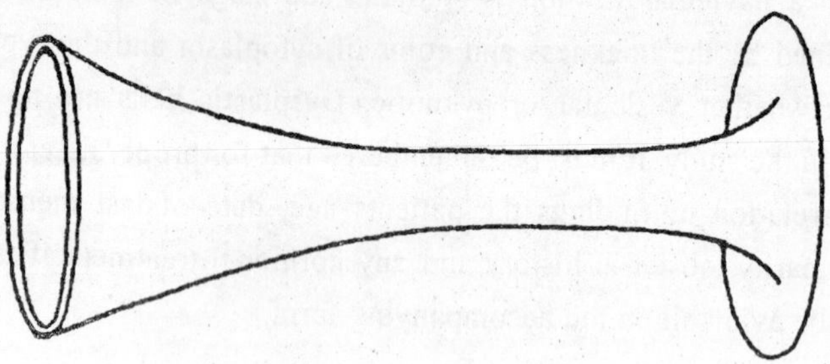

Figure 1.11 : Pinard's stethoscope

Technique

The wide end is placed over the patient's abdomen such that it is at right angle to the abdominal wall. The ear piece is applied near the ear and the instrument should not be touched by the hand while listening to the fetal heart. The maternal pulse is palpated at the same time to confirm that one is listening to the fetal heart and any maternal pulsations are not being wrongly transmitted. The probable site of finding the fetal heart is along the spino-umbilical line in vertex presentations. In case of breech it may be found at the level of the umbilicus or just above it while in a transverse lie the site depends on whether the fetus is placed dorso-inferior or dorso-superior.

BOULDELOQUE'S PELVIMETER

It is an instrument consisting of a pair of calipers and a measuring scale. It is designed to measure the external pelvic diameters, i.e. the diameters of the false pelvis. The measurement of these diameters helps in the assessment of the pelvic outlet and indicates to some extent the presence of gross cephalopelvic disproportion. The following diameters are measured:

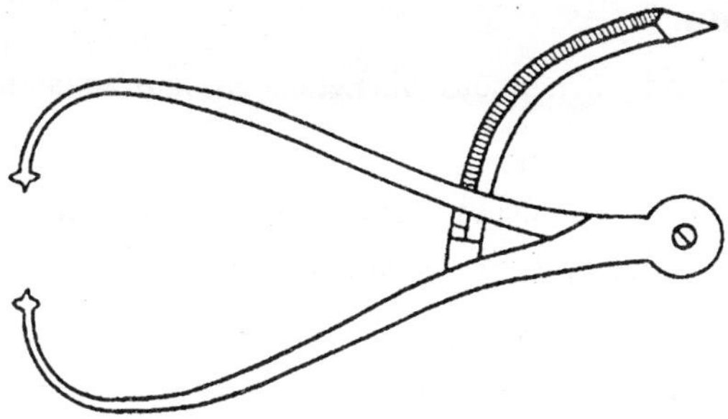

Figure 1.12 : Bouldeloque's pelvimeter

1. **External Conjugate :** It is the distance from the depression below the 5th lumbar spine to the upper border of symphysis pubis. It usually measures 8 inches.
2. **Interspinous diameter :** It is the distance between the two anterior superior iliac spines and measures about 10 inches.
3. **Intercristal diameter :** It is the distance between the outermost parts of both iliac crests and is around 11 inches.
4. **Intertrochanteric diameter :** It is the distance between the outer surfaces of the two greater trochanters and measures 12.5 inches.
5. **Obstetric Conjugate**

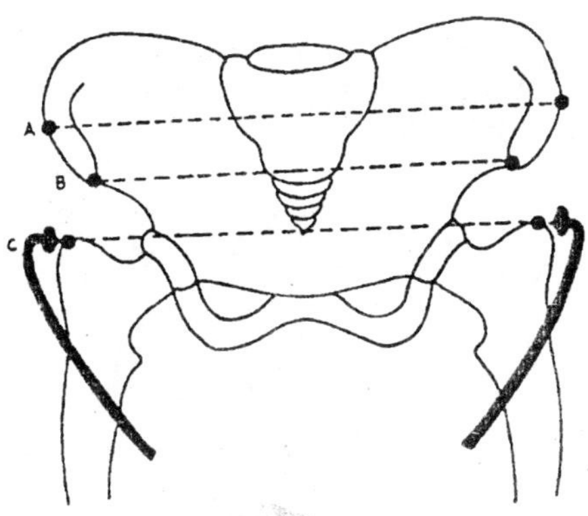

Figure 1.13 : Showing external pelvic diameters (a) Intercristal diameter, (b) Interspinous diameter, (c) Intertrochanteric diameter

Interpretation

1. Intercristal and interspinous diameters become equal in a flat pelvis.
2. Substraction of 3½ inches from external conjugate gives the approximate value of true conjugate.
3. When both intercristal and interspinous diameters are shortened it indicates a contracted pelvis.

Besides measuring the external diameters it can also predict the obstetric conjugate. The diagonal conjugate is the distance between the lower border of symphysis pubis to the upper border of sacral promontary.

Two fingers are introduced into the vagina and the sacral promontary is reached. The position where the lower border of symphysis pubis is falling on the hand is marked and the hand is withdrawn. The distance between the tip of the finger and the point marked on the hand is measured with the pelvimeter. This distance gives the diagonal conjugate. Substracting 1.5 cm from this gives the value of the obstetric conjugate. A value of less than 10 cm of obstetric conjugate indicates probable dystotia due to pelvic contraction.

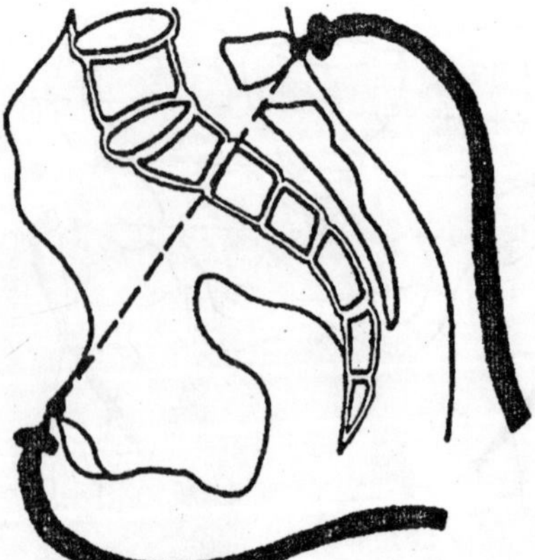

Figure 1.14 : Measurement of external conjugate

Chapter II

Instruments used in Dilatation, Curettage and Evacuation Operation (Including Medical Termination of Pregnancy)

HEGAR'S DILATORS

These instruments are sinuously curved double ended instruments and have conical tips. The tips are angled to the shaft and point in opposite directions. They are available in gradually increasing sizes ranging from a diameter of few millimeters to more than 2 cm. The dilators are numbered according to the diameter of the shaft. Two sizes are available in one double ended dilator with a difference of one mm. in their diameters.

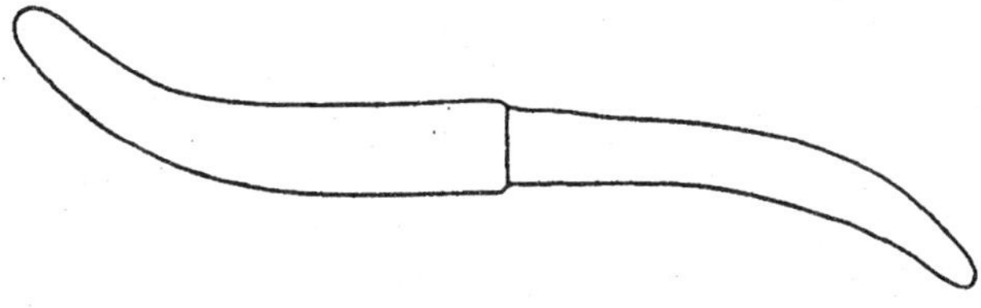

Figure 2.1 : Hegar's dilator

The operation can be done under general anaesthesia or sedation and paracervical block or only cervical block.

Technique

The patient is put in the lithotomy position and with full asepsis after retracting anterior and posterior vaginal walls and steadying the cervix with a volsellum the dilator is introduced in a pen holding manner. The ulnar border of the hand should rest against the patient's buttocks to prevent any injury from sudden and excessive dilatation. The dilator should be introduced keeping the tip directed anteriorly or posteriorly according to the direction of the uterus, whether anteverted or retroverted. The dilator should be introduced gently starting from a smaller size to gradually increasing sizes. If there is difficulty in dilatation or the cervix grips the dilator then the dilator is kept in position for sometime before introducing the next size.

For MTP operations the dilation required depends on size of the pregnancy, e.g. for 8 weeks size pregnancy dilatation should be upto number 8 dilator or just one size higher than that.

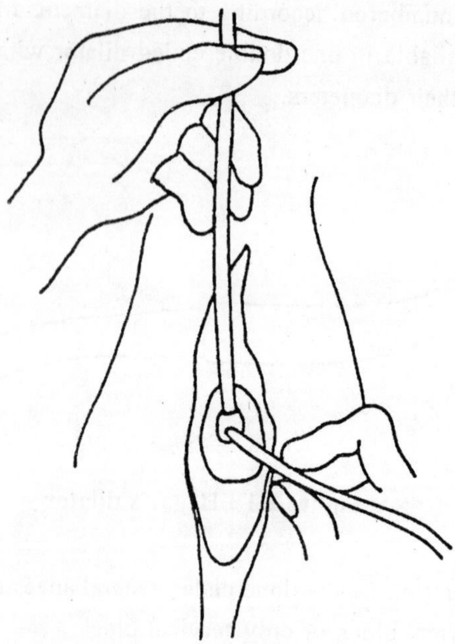

Figure 2.2 : Showing method of holding and introduction of dilator into the cervix.

Uses

I. Dilatation of the cervix is required in the following operations on uterine cavity in order to approach the uterine cavity.

1. In tubal insufflation test and HSG usually upto 5 mm. dilatation is required.
2. IUCD insertion may also require some amount of dilatation with number 4 and 5 dilators.
3. Prior to removing an endometrial polyp, placental polyp and fibroid polyp.
4. To reach the uterine cavity in endometrial biopsy, D & C, S & E and MTP. In MTP the dilatation required should be enough to allow easy passage and rotation of suction canula, i.e. for 8 mm suction canula No. 8 or 9 dilator may be used.
5. Prior to intracavitary radiotherapy.
6. During an elective LSCS or hysterotomy when the patient is not in labour and the os is closed, a dilator is used to dilate the cervix for drainage of lochia to prevent the formation of haematometra.
7. In Fothergill's repair to prevent cervical stenosis.
8. Prior to hysteroscopy.

II. Only dilatation is required in :

1. Hegar's test for incompetent cervical os: If No. 8 dilator is passed easily through the cervix without resistance then the cervix is incompetent and the test is positive.
2. Treatment of cervical stenosis.
3. In spasmodic dysmenorrhoea 25% patients are relieved when cervix is dilated upto No. 10 dilator.
4. Draining of haematometra and pyometra.
5. Prior to operations on cervix (e.g. repair operations, cautery, amputation etc.) to prevent stenosis.

III. Smaller sizes can also be used as urethral dilators.

Advantage

The angle makes the instrument less traumatic when used according to the direction of uterus. The gradually increasing sizes help in making the cervical canal patulous by stretching the muscle and fibrous tissue of the cervix without causing trauma and thus providing approach to the uterine cavity.

Disadvantage

The following complications may occur.

1. Sepsis, hemorrhage
2. Perforation
3. Cervical injuries.
4. Incompetent cervical os leading to habitual abortion or premature labour.
5. Injury to the bladder or rectum.

HAWKIN AMBLER'S DILATOR

This is a single ended cervical dilator with a circular flattened handle. The curvature is lesser than the Hegar's dilators. The technique, indications and complications are similar to those of Hegar's dilators.

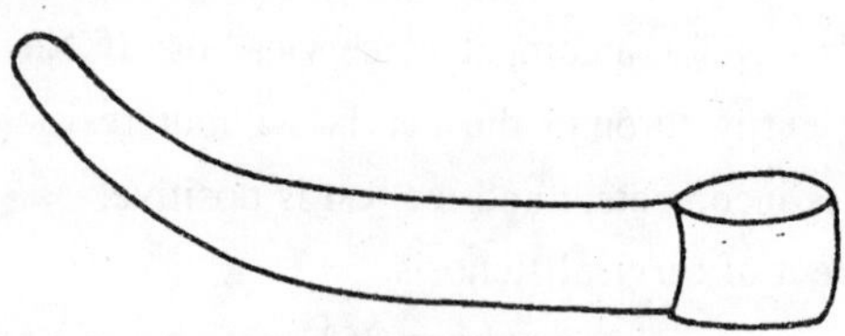

Figure 2.3 : Hawkin Ambler's dilator

RANDALL'S ENDOMETRIAL BIOPSY CURETTE

It is a slender hollow instrument with a stillete. The tip is blúnt and has a whistle subterminally. The whistle is notched and has a cutting edge. The instrument is angulated at about 5 cm from the tip so that it can be introduced according to the position of the uterus whether anteverted or retroverted in order to avoid perforations.

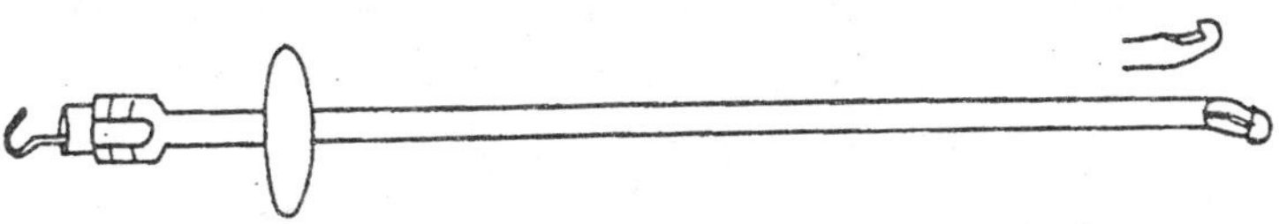

Figure 2.4 : Randall's endometrial biopsy curette

Technique

Endometrial biopsy is an outdoor procedure and usually requires no dilatation of the cervical canal. A local cervical block may be given and a sedative may be administered if the patient is apprehensive. The patency of the curette should be checked prior to use by flushing with normal saline. The curette is introduced with full asepsis after steadying the cervix with volsellum and retracting the anterior and posterior vaginal walls. It is brought in contact with the uterine walls and a strip of endometrium is removed with its cutting edge. Attaching a 10 ml syringe to the instrument to create small amount of negative pressure helps in sucking out the endometrial strip. The strip of tissue can be removed by flushing it out with air in a syringe. The tissue is sent in prelabelled vials for AFB culture and histopathology in normal saline and formalin respectively.

Uses

1. In cases of infertility for hormonal assessment. The tissue from isthmic region is not very sensitive to hormones, therefore care should be taken to avoid taking a specimen from this area in these cases. The timing is as follows:

(a) For diagnosis of anovulation tissue should be taken in secretary phase, i.e. one week prior to the menses in a regular 28 day cycle. If menses are irregular then it can be taken on the first day of the menses.

(b) For suspected corpus luteum insufficiency, ideally 2 biopsies should be taken on 21st and 24th day. If only one biopsy is possible then it maybe taken on the 24th day.

(c) In case of irregular ripening biopsy should be taken when menses start.

(d) In case of irregular shedding biopsy should be taken when menses stop but spotting continues.

2. In cases of primary or secondary amenorrhea.
3. Hormonal assessment in dysfunctional uterine bleeding.
4. Fractional curettage in suspected CA endometrium.
5. May be used for the removal of a missing IUCD in place of IUCD removing hook or for the removal of a tubal prosthesis after tuboplasty.

Disadvantages

1. Failure to obtain adequate amount of tissue.
2. Uterine perforation
3. Sepsis.

BLAKES' BLUNT AND SHARP UTERINE CURETTE

It is a long, double ended instrument. The terminal ends have oval loops which are angled to the shaft. One end has a sharp cutting edge while the other has a blunt edge. (compare with anterior vaginal wall retractor where the instrument is larger with transverse serrations on the loop). The curette comes in different sizes with the size of the loop varying from few millimeters to few centimeters. The sharp end has a smaller sized loop while blunt end has a larger loop.

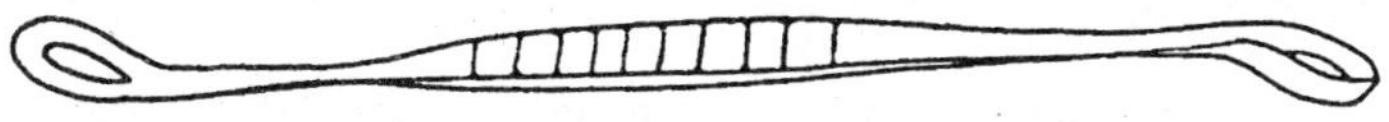

Figure 2.5 : Blakes' blunt and sharp uterine curette

Technique

The operation is done either under GA, or sedation and paracervical block. The instrument is introduced with full asepsis after retracting away posterior and anterior vaginal walls and steadying the cervix with a volsellum. The cervix is dilated by Hegar's dilator depending on the size of the curette and the indication of the operation. If the uterus is anteverted the curette is introduced with tip facing anteriorly while if it is retroverted it is introduced facing posteriorly to avoid perforation. The angulation between the loop and the shaft helps in easy removal of the uterine contents without causing injury to the uterus. The tissue is collected on a gauze piece, kept over the blade of the vaginal speculum and then sent for HPE and AFB culture as required.

Uses

A small sized uterine curette can be used in all the indications where endometrial biopsy curette is used.

I. Gynaecological Indications

Here the sharp end of the instrument is used.

1. Diagnosis of genital tuberculosis. The cornu should be specially curetted as genital tuberculosis starts from this area.
2. Infertility.
3. Dysfunctional uterine bleeding.
4. Primary and secondary amenorrhea

5. For fractional curettage in cases of CA endometrium and to assess the extent of uterine involvement in carcinoma cervix.

   Three specimens are taken and sent in labelled vials as follows:

   (a) Undilated endocervical canal.

   (b) Dilated cervix just above the internal os from isthmic region.

   (c) From uterine cavity (4 walls and fundus).

6. After removal of a uterine polyp and prior to myomectomy.
7. To diagnose causes of postmenopausal bleeding.
8. Treatment of Asherman's syndrome to break the adhesions.
9. Diagnosis of choriocarcinoma.

II. Obstetric indications

The blunt edge of the instrument is used for curetting the uterus in the following indications.

1. Incomplete abortion, medical termination of pregnancy by ovum forceps, for check curettage after S & E, operations and after evacuation for vesicular mole..
2. Check curettage in cases of postpartum hemorrhage to remove any retained products of conception.
3. Septic abortion.
4. Check curettage after vesicular mole evacuation may be done very gently.

Disadvantages

1. Sepsis
2. Hemorrhage
3. Over enthusiastic curettage can result in Asherman's syndrome leading to amenorrhea.
4. Infertility
5. Cervical injuries

LAMINARIA TENT

These are used as slow cervical dilators. They are made from *laminaria japonica*, a seaweed which is hygroscopic in nature. The stems of this weed are dried and cut into 6-8 cm pieces with diameters ranging from 2-10 mm. A string is looped through one end for ease of removal. The tents are sterilised prior to use. They swell up by 3-5 times of their size after absorbing the secretions of the cervical canal within 24 hours and thus dilate the cervix gradually and atraumatically. They are sterlized by ethylene oxide or by dipping in absolute alcohol.

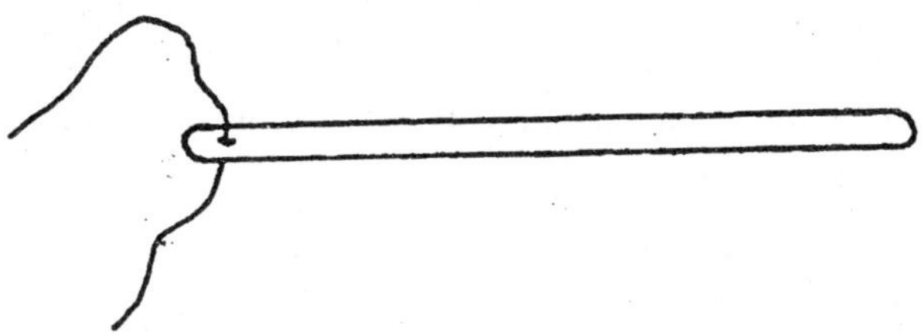

Figure 2.6 : Laminaria tent

Technique

The anterior and posterior vaginal walls are exposed and the cervix is grasped with a volsellum. The uterine cavity is sounded to know the length of the cervical canal and the level of the internal os. The tent is then passed to lie just beyond the internal os. One or more laminaria tents may be needed to fit smugly into the cervical canal. The vagina may be packed with sterile gauge after fixing the terminal ends of the tent to the gauze. This prevents premature expulsion and makes it easier to remove them. They may be removed after 24 hours and a second set may be inserted if dilatation is not adequate.

Uses

1. First trimester and second trimester pregnancy termination.
2. Induction of labour

Advantage

They dilate the cervix gradually, so there are minimal chances of injury to the cervix and any late sequelae like incompetent cervical os is prevented.

Disadvantages

1. Infection
2. Dumbbell formation: When it is placed too high above the os it swells up unequally. The supracervical portion swells up more than the cervical portion making its removal difficult and may at times require hysterotomy.
3. If tip lies below the os its purpose is wasted and the os remains undilated.
4. Migration upwards into the uterine cavity may occur.
5. False passage may be created during insertion.

LAMINARIA TENT INTRODUCING FORCEPS

It is a long forceps with 2 blades, a joint, shank and handles with a lock. The forceps is angled near the blades and the blades are deeply grooved to hold a tubular structure. When apposed together it used to introduce the laminaria tents into the cervical canal.

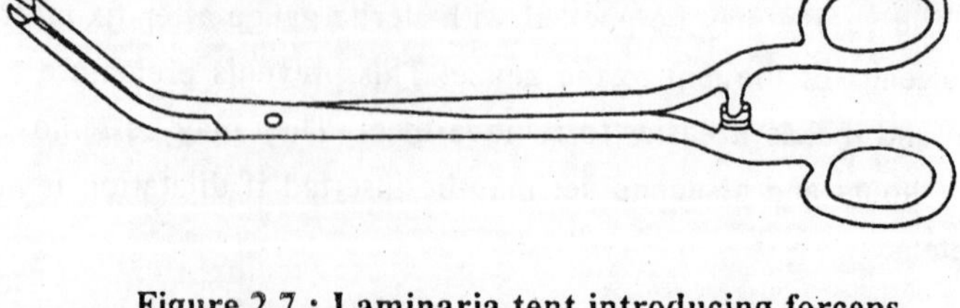

Figure 2.7 : Laminaria tent introducing forceps

HAYWOOD SMITH'S OVUM FORCEPS

It is a long straight instrument with 2 spoon shaped blades, a shank and a hand. There is no lock in this instrument. The spoon shaped blades have multiple longitudinal fenestrations and are well apposed when closed. The blades can hold a good amount of tissue in between. The absence of a lock minimises damage to any structure which may be accidently held in between the blades.

The forceps is available with varying sizes of blades used according to the necessity, the larger one for advanced pregnancies and smaller one for early pregnancies. The fenestrations allow part of the tissue to bulge out so that the grip is secure.

Technique

The operation may be done under GA, sedation or paracervical block.. With full asepsis the anterior and posterior vaginal walls are retracted away and the cervix is steadied with a volsellum. If not already dilated the cervical canal is dilated and the required size of the ovum forceps is introduced with the blades closely approximated. Once inside the uterine cavity the blades are opened up and the products of conception are grasped. The forceps is withdrawn after a few gentle rotatory movements which help in detaching the products of conception from the uterus.

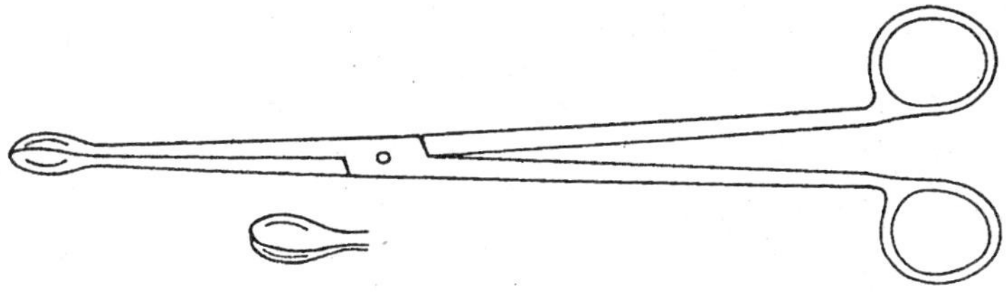

Figure 2.8 : Haywood Smith's ovum forceps

Uses

1. To remove the products of conception in :
   (a) Ist trimester pregnancy termination.
   (b) Incomplete abortion.
   (c) Septic abortion.
2. To explore the uterine cavity for placental bits and membranes in PPH.
3. Removal of a foreign body from the uterus (e.g. septic abortion).

Disadvantages

1. Perforation
2. Sepsis
3. Injury to intra-abdominal structures like bowel, omentum etc. secondary to uterine perforation.
4. Incomplete evacuation.

KARMAN'S DOUBLE WHISTLE SUCTION CANULA

It is a long tubular structure made of either plastic or metal. The instrument may be either straight or slightly angulated. The distal end is double–whistled subterminally while the proximal end fixes into the tubing of the suction apparatus. Each whistle has a superior overhanging edge which acts as a curette. The proximal end is attached to an adaptor arrangement with a hole which when covered with the thumb and connected to the suction apparatus creates a negative pressure. When the thumb is removed the vacuum is broken. The sizes available vary from number 4 to 16. The number of the canula corresponds to the diameter of the canula in millimeters. The plastic canula may be of rigid or flexible type. The plastic type is superior since it is disposable, less traumatic and transparent so that the contents being evacuated are visible.

Figure 2.9 : Karman's double whistle suction canula

Technique

The operation can be done under GA, sedation and cervical block or only cervical block. The anterior and posterior walls are retracted away and cervix is steadied with a volsellum with full asepsis. The cervix is first dilated with gradually increasing sizes of Hegar's dilators. The dilatation should be just enough to allow easy passage and rotation of the canula, e.g. No. 8 or 9 Hegar's dilator for a 8 mm size canula. The size of the canula chosen should be equal to the size of gestation in weeks (No. 8 canula for a 8 weeks pregnancy). The canula is initially inserted only upto the level of the lower segment of the uterus. The thumb is placed over the hole to create a negative pressure after the suction is switched on. The canula is rotated along all the walls of the uterine cavity. Strong in and out movements of the canula are not required as this may cause perforation. When the uterus is emptied and air bubbles are visible in the canula, it is removed but only after breaking the vacuum by first removing the thumb from the hole. A check curettage may be done to confirm that the evacuation is complete.

The following signs suggest complete evacuation :

(a) Uterus grips the canula
(b) Bleeding stops
(c) Uterus contracts and appears firm.
(d) Bubbles appear
(e) Uterine walls give a gritty feeling on check curettage.

The operation is incomplete unless the aspirated contents are examined to confirm evacuation so that ectopic pregnancy and hydatid mole are ruled out. Pregnancies beyond 9 weeks have recognisable fetal parts while early pregnancies can be washed and put in glass container in water when chorionic villi appear as soft, fluffy, feathery finger-like projections. A simple magnifying glass may be used to confirm their presence. If the patient is Rh negative, 50 μgm of anti-D immunoglobulin should be administered.

Uses

1. In medical termination of pregnancy.
2. Suction and evacuation of vesicular mole.
3. S and E of incomplete abortion.
4. S & E of missed abortion.
5. May be used for draining out brain matter and CSF after craniotomy for a hydrocephalic baby or cephalopelvic disproportion with dead baby.

Disadvantages

The complications are rare but following may occur.

1. Cervical injuries
2. Uterine perforations
3. Cervical incompetence
4. Hemorrhage
5. Sepsis
6. Ashermann's syndrome.
7. Injury to bladder, bowel, omentum, etc.

SORRENSON'S PLASTIC SUCTION CANULA

The technique and indications of use are similar to Karman's canula. The only difference is in the shape as here the canula has only a single whistle which is present subterminally while Karman's type has double whistles.

Figure 2.10 : Sorrenson's plastic suction canula

KARMAN'S MENSTRUAL REGULATION SYRINGE

This instrument is used for aspiration of uterine contents within 14 days of a missed period, i.e. 44 days of the last menstrual period. This operation is known as menstrual aspiration, menstrual induction, instant period, atraumatic abortion, mini abortion, besides menstrual regulation. It is a 50 ml reusable plastic syringe fitted to a 4-6 mm plastic canula. It has a rubber syringe and a piston which does not get detached during intense suction because of presence of an internal lock. Flared outside arms are present to hold the syringe in the extended position. There is a pressure control valve at the end of the nozzle. The piston has a finger grip for convenience of use. Though disposable, it can perform upto 40 MR operations after sterilisation if used carefully.

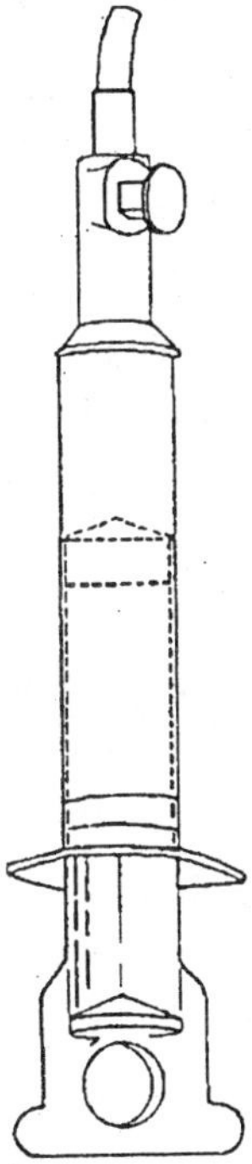

Figure 2.11 : Karman's menstrual regulation syringe

Technique

It is an outdoor procedure but paracervical block is required.

SIMPSON'S MODIFICATION OF OLDHAM'S PERFORATOR

It is used in craniotomy to enter the fetal skull and collapse it by draining out the brain matter. It consists of a blade about 1 inch. in length having an inner blunt and an outer cutting edge, a shoulder just below the blades, a shank and a handle with metal bars. The metal bars help in maintaining a rigid fixation of the handles keeping the blades in close approximation when the head is being pierced.

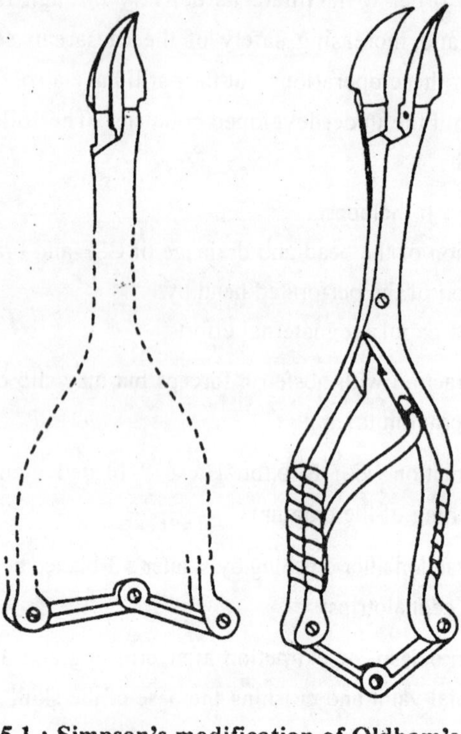

Figure 5.1 : Simpson's modification of Oldham's perforator

Indications of craniotomy

1. Live baby with hydrocephalus
2. Dead baby with,
   (a) forecoming head with cephalopelvic disproportion

The procedure is done with full asepsis. The anterior and posterior vaginal walls are retracted away and the cervix is grasped with a volsellum. The canula is introduced inside the uterine cavity after closing the valve. The piston is drawn out till it gets locked and a pressure of 60 cm of H_2O is created in the syringe. The valve is now opened and uterine aspiration starts with gentle rotatory movements. When the syringe fills upto 25-30 ml, it is emptied and reintroduced as before. It must be remembered that the valve should be closed before withdrawing the syringe. Also, the piston should never be thrust forwards while the canula is within the uterine cavity as it may cause air embolism. The process is repeated till the uterus is emptied and a gritty feeling is obtained indicative of complete evacuation.

Advantages

1. No anaesthesia is needed.
2. No psychological trauma of termination to the patient.
3. Procedure is inexpensive.
4. Procedure is independent of electric supply which is a problem in developing and underdeveloped areas.
5. Instrument can be easily transported.
6. Relatively simple procedure.

Disadvantages

1. The procedure may be performed on a non-pregnant lady with some other cause of delayed menses rather than pregnancy.
2. It may fail to aspirate a high implanted zygote.
3. Ectopic pregnancy may be missed.
4. Rarely can cause cervical or uterine injuries.
5. Cannot be used for uterine sizes of more than 8 weeks.
6. Hemorrhage may occur as the process of evacuation is slow.
7. Sepsis may result.

Chapter III

Instruments for Tubal Patency Tests

RUBIN'S TUBAL INSUFFLATION TEST AND HYSTEROSALPINGOGRAPHY CANULA

It is a curved hollow tube with multiple side apertures near the tip. A conical rubber collar is fitted 5-6 cm behind the tip of the tube which presses against the external os after the canula has been introduced inside the uterine cavity preventing back leakage of the air during insufflation. A rubber tubing connects the open end of the canula to the CO_2 delivery or the air delivery apparatus.

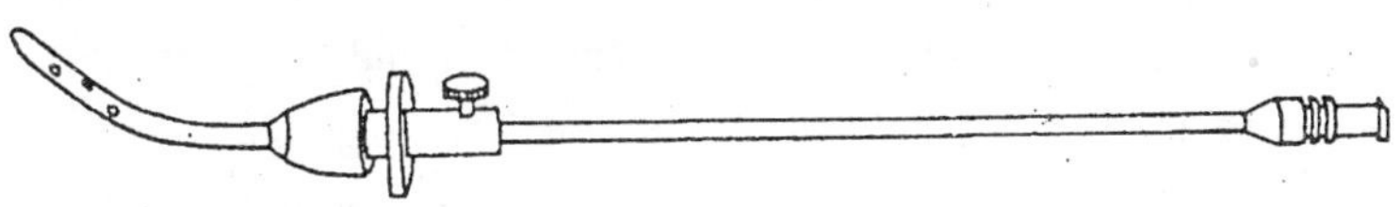

Figure 3.1: Rubin's tubal insufflation canula

Uses

1. Tubal insufflation test
2. Hysterosalpingography
3. Laparoscopic chromopertubation
4. Hydrotubations

I. Tubal Insufflation Test

Technique

The test is done in cases of infertility to test the patency of the fallopian tubes. The test has both diagnostic and therapeutic advantages. It is performed just after menses because in the second half of the cycle it may disturb an implanted zygote. The canula should be flushed to check its patency prior to its use to avoid a false negative test. CO_2 is used for insufflation as it is highly soluble in blood so there are lesser chances of embolism if it enters the blood stream through uterine sinuses. The CO_2 gas is supplied at a steady flow rate through a delivery system having a safety valve which maintains a pressure less than 200 mm Hg. The pressure recordings are made on a revolving drum by a Kymograph.

This is an outpatient procedure not requiring anaesthesia or analgesia unless the patient is apprehensive. Inj. Atropine is given to the patient prior to operation. A per vaginum examination is done to know the size and position of the uterus and to rule out local infection and pelvic inflammatory disease. The anterior and posterior vaginal walls are retracted away and the cervix is grasped with a tenaculum. The canula is introduced directly or after dilatation with No. 4 or 5 Hegar's dilator if needed. The other end of the canula is connected to the CO_2 delivery system and Kymograph apparatus. The conical rubber collar should fit snugly over the external os to prevent leakage of the gas. This is achieved by pulling the cervix over the rubber collar by the tenaculum. The CO_2 is now delivered at a steady flow rate of 60 ml/min and pressures are recorded on the Kymograph.

Results and their interpretation

(a) If one or both the tubes are patent there is an initial rise of pressure to 60 mm Hg followed by a wave pattern horizontal tracing indicating tubal peristalsis. Clinically passage of air from the tubes to the peritoneal cavity may be auscultated over lower abdomen as a bubbling or squeaking sound. The patient also experiences pain on the shoulder when the gas comes under the diaphragm. A plain

X-ray abdomen may demonstrate a crescentic shadow below the diaphragm indicating presence of air.

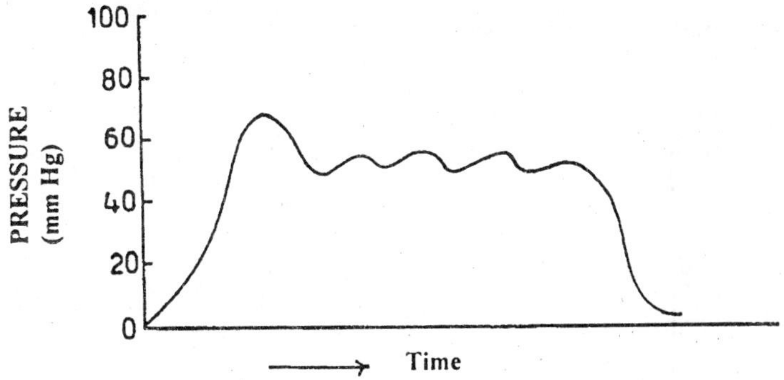

Figure 3.2 : Normal tubal insufflation curve showing wave pattern

(b) Peritubal adhesions due to previous salpingitis prevents normal peristaltic action of the tubes. The initial pressure rise is high upto 150-200 mm Hg and is followed by a smooth descending pattern in these cases, as opposed to the normal wave pattern. This indicates tubal patency without peristalsis.

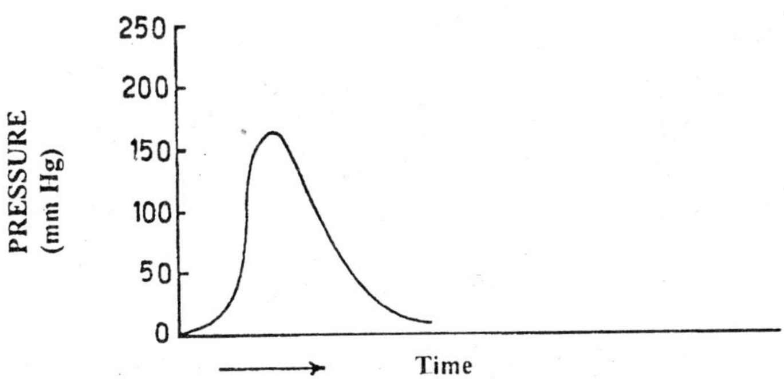

Figure 3.3 : Abolition of wave pattern in peritubal adhesions

(c) In case there is no true block but the tubes are in a state of spasm there is a rapid rise of pressure to 150-200 mm Hg followed by descending pattern when the safety valve opens up. This pattern can be abolished by the administration of amylnitrite and a normal curve is obtained after the spasm is relieved.

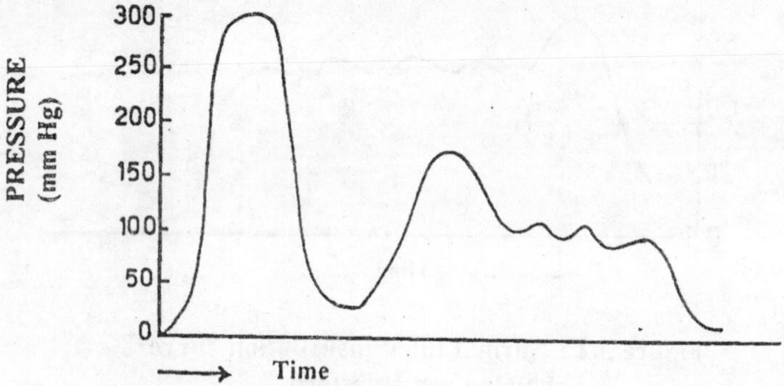

Figure 3.4 : Tubal spasm relieved by amyl nitrite

(d) In case of tubal occlusion the gas fails to pass into the peritoneal cavity and even after administration of amylnitrite the same findings are obtained, i.e. a sudden increase upto 150-200 mm Hg followed by a sudden decrease due to opening of the safety valve.

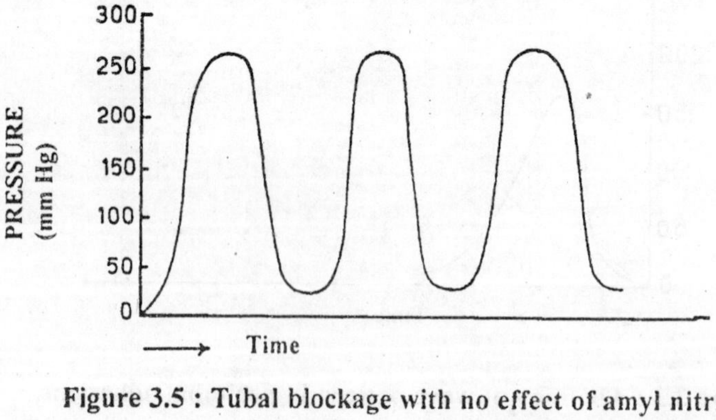

Figure 3.5 : Tubal blockage with no effect of amyl nitrite

Following points should be remembered while interpreting the results :

1. If insufflation test fail on at least two occasions only then should the tubes be pronounced as blocked.
2. False positive readings are sometimes obtained owing to back leakage of gas or accumulation of air in a large hydrosalpinx even when the tubes are blocked.
3. False negative results may be obtained if the tubes are in spasm.

Advantages

The test is a cheap, simple, outpatient procedure to detect tubal blockage in cases of infertility.

Disadvantages

1. Pelvic inflammatory disease may flare up.
2. Patient may have severe pain and collapse due to vasovagal shock.
3. An early pregnancy may be dislodged if timing is not immediately after menses.
4. Patient can die due to embolism. It is this risk which has made the procedure obsolete and other techniques are now being preferred.

II. Hysterosalpingography

This is a procedure where the uterine cavity and the fallopian tubes are visualised after pushing a radio opaque dye through a Rubin's canula. The procedure is visualised over an image intensifier and radiographs may be taken for a permanent record.

Technique

Timing of the investigation is immediately after menstruation so that the risk of dislodging an implanted zygote is ruled out. Any local infection and pelvic inflammatory disease are contra-indications to the procedure. The procedure does not require anaesthesia or analgesia unless the patient is very apprehensive. Inj. Atropine should be administered half hour before the procedure and patient may be given analgesics e.g. tab Brufen 600 mg in the morning.

The vaginal walls are retracted away and cervix is grasped with a tenaculum. The canula is introduced inside the uterine cavity and is made to fit snugly over it to prevent leakage. The uterus is anteverted so that the tubes do not lie posteriorly and the passage of dye into tubes and then into the peritoneal cavity is better visualised. The dye used may be oil based e.g. lipidiol or water soluble. Water soluble dyes are safer as there are lesser chances of embolism if accidently pushed into the blood stream via open uterine sinuses. Other advantage is that these are less irritant with lesser chances of inflammatory reaction and adhesion formation in the pelvis. Also there is a lesser incidence of hypersensitivity reaction with these. However, the fat soluble dyes give a better visualisation as they are absorbed slowly giving a better contrast. The incidence of inflammatory reactions, adhesion formation and hypersensitivity is higher alongwith the danger of embolism in fat soluble dyes.

About 10-15 ml of the dye is gently pushed inside the uterine cavity through the canula and any back leakage is checked. The dye is seen to fall into the peritoneal cavity through the fallopian tube ostia over an image intensifier and X-rays are taken for a permanent record. The maximum screening time should not be more than 30 sec. and more than 2 X-ray pictures should not be taken to minimise radiation damage to the female gonad.

Uses

1. To demonstrate tubal anatomy, function and site of block.
2. To diagnose any suspected congenital uterine anomaly e.g.:
   (a) bicornuate uterus

(b) subseptate uterus

(c) arcuate uterus.

3. To diagnose the site, size and mechanical changes in the shape of the uterus from a space occupying lesion e.g. submucous fibroid.
4. To demonstrate cervical incompetence when radiograph will show funneling of the cervical canal..
5. To assess the success of tuboplasty operation.

Advantage

The advantage of this test over the tubal insufflation test is that though expensive it gives a wider spectrum of information besides recording the results permanently for future reference.

Disadvantages

The test is expensive and following complications may result:

1. Pelvic inflammatory disease may flare up.
2. Patient may collapse and have severe pain.
3. Allergic reactions, even anaphylaxis may result.
4. An early pregnancy maybe dislodged.
5. In case of fat soluble dye embolism may occur.

III. Laparoscopic chromopertubation

Here methylene blue dye is pushed via the canula from the cervix and the appearance of the dye from the fimbrial end is visualised by a laparoscope. The advantage is that tubal status as well as peritoneal factors contributing to infertility can be assessed at the same sitting.

IV. Tubal Patency by Ultra Sonography

The amount of fluid in pouch of Doughlas is measured followed by injection of normal saline through HSG canula. Increase in amount of fluid in POD indicates patency besides direct visualisation of fluid spurting out from fimbrial end as the 'waterfall' sign.

Contra indications to tubal patency tests

1. If patient is in post ovulatory period.
2. In the presence of pelvic inflammatory disease.
3. Patient is sensitive to iodine or any of the ingredients of the dye.

Chapter IV

Obstetric Forceps and Ventouse

OBSTETRIC FORCEPS

It is an instrument designed to hold the fetal head to effect a speedy delivery during the second stage of labour.

History

The instrument was first used in a very crude form in the 17th century by the Chamberlain family in England. The technique was kept a secret and was discovered only in the 18th century. Palfyn was the first obstetrician to describe this instrument in 1720. The earlier instruments were either metallic or wooden and consisted of straight blades joined together with a handle. The straight blades could grip the head only behind the center of the pelvic axis. As the pelvic canal is curved forwards the following disadvantages were seen :

(a) It increased the extension at the neck, as it could grip the head behind the center. This resulted in larger diameters of the head coming into play.

(b) A large amount of force was misdirected.

(c) The soft parts between the fetal head and the symphysis pubis were crushed.

Subsequent modifications were made to improve its design. Leveret in 1751, introduced the pelvic curve. Later, Smellie introduced the shanks so that the instrument became longer and the forceps could be locked under vision even when the head was high up. Tarnier in 1877 introduced the axis traction rods which pulled the head along the axis of the pelvic canal and thus lesser force was now required to deliver the head. The forceps became lighter and any injury from it was of lesser degree.

Description

The instrument consists of 2 branches with the following parts:

1. Two blades each having a pelvic curve and a cephalic curve.
2. Shanks
3. Handles
4. Lock: The lock may be of 2 types:

(a) Sliding lock : The sliding lock as in Kjelland's forceps consists of a single U-shaped receptacle mounted midway on the left shank which accepts the shank of the right blade. The sliding lock allows the blades to move forwards and backwards independently and can help in delivering the baby by asynclitism.

(b) Fixed lock : It may be of English type or French type. English lock is commoner and consists of a socket located on the shank at its junction with the handle which fits into a similarly located socket on the opposite shank. The French lock consists of a threaded bolt screwed into a hole in the left shank. A notch in the right shank articulates with this bolt. After each blade has been applied to the fetal head the notch is moved over the eye bolt and the bolt is tightened to lock the blades firmly together.

Types and classification of forceps operation

I. Depending on the station of the head

1. Outlet forceps operation : The fetal head has reached the perineal floor, the scalp is visible between contractions and the head has rotated in the antero-posterior diameter or is within 45° of the midline.

2. Low forceps operation : Biparietal diameter has crossed the level of the ischial spines but not reached the perineal floor and rotation is not complete.

3. Mid forceps operation : When the biparietal diameter of fetal head has entered the pelvic brim but is at or above the level of the ischial spines. It has two subvarieties.

(a) **High mid forceps :** The biparietal diameter has crossed the pelvic brim but is above the level of ischial spines.

(b) **Low mid forceps operation :** The biparietal diameter has crossed the brim and is lying at the level of the ischial spines.

4. **High Forceps operation :** Here the biparietal diameter has not crossed the pelvic brim. This type of forceps application is obsolete owing to serious maternal injuries inflicted during the operation.

II. Depending on Type of Application

1. **Cephalic application :** The application is in relation to the biparietal diameter and the grip is mento-occipital. It is a safe and secure grip which causes least injury to the baby as the blades are applied directly in relation to the baby's head irrespective of the maternal diameters. However, this may lead to gross maternal injuries during delivery unless the forceps used has a negligible pelvic curve.

2. **Pelvic application :** Here the forceps is applied correctly in relation to the pelvis such that the blades are placed parallel to the pelvic axis irrespective of the position of the head. This type of application can cause gross injuries to the fetal head and can be successful only when the fetal head is in the antero-posterior diameter.

3. **Ideal application :** When the pelvic and cephalic application of the forceps correspond with each other the operation is most successful and safe.

Indications for obstetric forceps

I. Conditions threatening the life of the mother

1. Severe preeclamptic toxemia.
2. Eclampsia.
3. Pregnancy with heart disease
4. Pregnancy with pulmonary disease, e.g. bronchial asthma.
5. Pregnancy with chronic renal disease

6. Pregnancy with severe anaemia.
7. Maternal distress.

II. Dangers threatening the life of the baby

1. Foetal distress.
2. Cord prolapse
3. Prematurity
4. Meconium stained liquor.

III. Prolonged second stage of labour

1. Faults in the forces
   - (a) incoordinate uterine action
   - (b) impending uterine inertia
   - (c) epidural block, anaesthetics, analgesics
   - (d) poor maternal effort
2. Faults in the passage
   - (a) tight perineum
   - (b) mild cephalopelvic disproportion
3. Faults in the passenger
   - (a) after coming head of breech
   - (b) face with mentoanterior position
   - (c) persistent occipitoposterior, deep transverse arrest
   - (d) large baby

Technique of the forceps operation

The following are the prerequisites for a successful forceps application.

1. Full aseptic precautions should be taken
2. The position of the patient should be lithotomy or left lateral.
3. Bowel and bladder should be empty.
4. Anaesthetist and paediatrician should be present.
5. Patient should be fully prepared for cesarean section in case the forceps application fails, e.g. in difficult cases .

6. The cervix should be fully dilated
7. The membranes should be ruptured
8. The head should be engaged, i.e. the biparietal diameter should have crossed the pelvic brim.
9. The uterus should be actively contracting and relaxing.
10. The head should be rotated and should lie in the antero-posterior diameter.
11. Episiotomy, if needed should be given.
12. The presentation should be vertex or face with mento-anterior or aftercoming head of breech.
13. There should not be any gross cephalopelvic disproportion.
14. Consent should be taken.

I. The Low Forceps Operation & Outlet Forceps Operation

This operation is done when the maximum diameter of the head is below the ischial spines with the head resting on the perineum. A short forceps or a light weight long curved forceps is used, e.g. Wriggleys forceps. The head is usually lying in the anteroposterior diameter with the rotation completed. However, deficient rotation can be completed by rotating manually before the blades are applied. The forceps is applied parallel to the pelvic axis such that it grips the biparietal diameter of the head in the mento-occipital axis. The operation is completed in two steps. Prior to application the prerequisites as described above should be checked and a pudendal block should be given.

(a) Application of the blades

The forceps is assembled in the correct anatomical position so that the cephalic curve is facing inwards and pelvic curve facing upwards. When so placed the left blade is in the left hand of the surgeon while the right blade is in the right hand of the surgeon. The left blade is applied first. It is held in a pen-holding manner and introduced parallel to the opposite ilioinguinal ligament after protecting the vagina with the fingers of the right hand. The blade is pushed up between the fetal head and the sacral hollow and then swept up such that it comes to lie on the left side of the pelvis. The right blade is then introduced in a similar manner and then both the blades are locked during contraction. Failure of the blades to lock indicates incomplete rotation.

(b) Extraction of the head

Following points have to be remembered for a safe extraction of the baby.

1. To extract the head slowly and gently.
2. To pull during a uterine contraction and wait in between.
3. To unlock the blades in between uterine contractions in order to prevent injury to the baby from prolonged, continuous pressure.
4. To direct the pulls along the axis of the pelvic canal depending on the station of the head.

Thus to extract the baby the head should be pulled after locking the blades during a good uterine contraction. The direction of the pull should be first downwards towards the patient's feet and then gradually forwards towards patient's abdomen and finally upwards towards the head end of the patient to deliver the head by extension. The instrument is gripped by the right hand and delivery of the head is completed by pulling in the above directions. The blades of the forceps are now removed in the opposite order, right blade is removed first and left blade is removed next.

II. The Midforceps Operation

Here the forceps is applied for the delivery of the head which is at or above the level of the ischial spines and has crossed the pelvic brim. The long curved forceps, e.g. Haigh Ferguson's forceps or the Kjelland's forceps with wandering method of application may be chosen. Most of these are cases of persistent occipitoposterior or deep transverse arrest. There is not much difference between these and the low forceps operation except that here the malrotation has to be corrected first and GA is needed as the head in this case lies at a higher level. The blades have to be inserted higher up with more chances of infection and injuries. The direction of pull is first backwards, then downwards, forwards and upwards. The operation is more difficult and liable to complications.

FORCEPS APPLICATION IN DIFFICULT SITUATIONS

I. The High Forceps Operation

The high forceps operation is now obsolete. It was done when the maximum diameter of the head was above the pelvic brim. There are three methods of application:

1. Classical or indirect method

This was the oldest method of application. The blades were applied with the cephalic curve facing the symphysis pubis until it reached the neck of the fetus and then it was rotated by 180°. The posterior blade was applied next and the baby was delivered. The above method has been discarded as it caused severe maternal injuries.

2. Direct method

Here the anterior blade of the forceps was applied directly to the fetal head by cephalic application of the forceps. The posterior blade was applied through the sacrum and baby delivered by traction. This method also caused fetal and maternal injuries so was discarded.

3. Wandering method

Here in order to minimise maternal injuries both the blades are applied through the sacral hollow which has more space. The forceps is articulated and kept in its correct anatomical position with the knob on the shank pointing towards the occiput of the baby. The blade which now lies towards anterior side of the patient, i.e. towards her abdomen is the anterior blade. There are 3 principles of application :

(a) Anterior blade is applied first.

(b) Knob on the shank of the forceps faces the occiput of the baby.

(c) The occiput has to be brought anteriorly by rotating it with the forceps.

The anterior blade is passed through the sacral hollow after protecting maternal tissues with a gloved hand. It is rotated and swept across the baby's face and brought to lie anteriorly. The posterior blade is now applied from the sacral hollow and the forceps is locked. The occiput is rotated and brought anteriorly and the head is delivered by traction.

II. Forceps Operation in the Occipitoposterior Position

The occiput lies in the hollow of the sacrum with the maximum transverse diameter lying at or above the level of the ischial spines. The following methods may be used.

1. The method of choice is manual rotation of the head with forceps extraction as in mid forceps delivery.
2. Alternatively axis traction apparatus maybe used which does not require prior rotation of the head because the ball and socket joint in the traction handle allows the instrument and the head to rotate together. The blades are removed when anterior rotation has occurred and reapplied in the usual way to extract the head.
3. Forceps rotation and forceps delivery with a Kjellands forceps may be done by 'wandering method' or a 'double application technique' or 'Scanzoni's manoeuvre' may be used with any mid cavity forceps. In the first application the blades are applied as in a cephalic application, i.e. correctly in relation to the fetal head irrespective of the pelvis. The occiput is then rotated anteriorly which makes the blades inverted so that the pelvic curve faces downwards. The blades

are removed and reapplied as in a pelvic application parallel to the walls of the pelvis. The baby is extracted by pulling backwards, downwards, forwards and then upwards. (Figure 4.5)

4. When the occiput is directly posterior the blades can be applied without rotation and a pelvic application is done. The direction of pull in this face to pubes delivery is backwards, downwards until the occiput descends down and the root of the nose abuts against the symphysis pubis. The occiput is then delivered by pulling forwards until it slips over the perineum when the direction of pull is changed to backwards and downwards to deliver the forehead and the face.

III. Forceps Operation in Face Presentation

This is attempted only in mento-anterior positions. The blades are applied to the well-rotated head by a pelvic application as in case of a vertex position in the mento-occipital axis. Care should be taken to avoid injury to the eyes of the baby. The direction of pull is backwards, downwards until the chin comes to rest against the symphysis pubis. The forceps is now raised forwards and upwards to deliver the face, forehead, vertex and the occiput by flexion.

IV. Forceps Operation in aftercoming Head of Breech

This operation may be completed by an ordinary long forceps when the breech has delivered and the head is long delayed in the pelvic cavity. The operation is not attempted in an unengaged head. If the occiput is anterior the body of the baby is held forwards against the mother's abdomen and forceps are applied prefably below it but can be applied infront of it also. The direction of pull is backwards, downwards, forwards and upwards. When the occiput is posterior the forceps should be applied in front of the body of the baby which is allowed to hang down.

V. Forceps Application in Contracted Pelvis

It has limited use in a contracted pelvis and the operation should only be a tentative trial of forceps, i.e., if the head moves down with a few pulls of moderate force the traction may be continued otherwise one should opt for a cesarean section. The rule is to put the patient under general anaesthesia and then assess the pelvis, the size of the head, the station, amount of moulding and then decide for the route of delivery. The forceps can compress the biparietal diameter by 1 cm Excessive compression is harmful for the baby.

VI. Failed forceps operation

It denotes an unsuccessful attempt to deliver with forceps. Failure may be due to the inability to apply the blades or an inability to deliver the baby after the blades have been applied. The causes may be either a failure of application or of extraction.

1. Application of blades to an unrotated head.
2. Incompletely dilated cervix.
3. Cephalopelvic disproportion.
4. Presence of a contraction ring in the uterus above the level of the fetal head.
5. Fetal anomaly, e.g. hydrocephalus; conjoined twins

VII. Prophylactic Forceps

It is the application of forceps before any of the three primary indications ie maternal distress, foetal distress or prolonged second stage have arisen. It is applied in anticipation of these problems to cut short avoidable discomfort and stress. It should not be taken as a license for meddlesome midwifery and should be attempted only when safe forceps delivery is likely to occur and should be avoided if the delivery is likely to be dangerous and difficult.

MECHANISM OF ACTION OF THE OBSTETRIC FORCEPS

1. **Traction :** The action is essentially one of pull on the fetal head, e.g. in cases of inadequate uterine contractions, poor maternal effort, mild cephalopelvic disproportion.

2. **Head compression** : This occurs to some extent and ensures a firm grip. The biparietal diameter can be reduced upto 8.4 cm and this helps in negotiating mild disproportion. It must be remembered however that excessive compression of the head may cause intracranial disturbances and result in the baby being born in a state of asphyxia.

3. **Rotation** : Forceps is used for rotating the head as in the case of persistent occipitoposterior position or deep transverse arrest in order to bring the sagittal suture in the antero-posterior diameter of the pelvis. This may however result in maternal injuries.

4. **Lateral lever action** : This type of action may sometimes be used by carrying the blades gently from side to side and making use of available space in order to deliver the baby. But it is avoided because of risk of maternal injury.

5. **Stimulation of uterus** : The forceps is said to increase the force and intensity of the uterine contractions to some extent though the mechanism is unknown.

Complications of Forceps Operations

The following maternal and fetal complications may result :

1. Sepsis
2. Complications associated with anaesthesia.
3. Maternal injuries.
   (a) tears of the perineum
   (b) tears of the cervix
   (c) tears of the vagina.
   (d) rupture of the uterus.
4. Injury to rectum or bladder
5. Post partum hemorrhage which may be atonic type or may be due to maternal injuries.
6. Intracranial hemorrhages in the baby specially if the blades are applied in the occipitofrontal diameter of the head.

7. Depressed fractures of the skull.
8. Tears of the tentorium cerebelli.
9. Asphyxia from cerebral compression.
10. Nerve injuries, e.g., VII nerve palsy; Brachial plexus injury.
11. Cephalohaematoma.

DESCRIPTION OF INDIVIDUAL FORCEPS

KJELLAND'S FORCEPS

It is a long straight forceps introduced in 1916. The use of this forceps is now obsolete however it is only very rarely used in persistent occipito-posterior positions. The forceps has a cephalic curve and negligible pelvic curve. The length is 15.5 inches and the maximum distance between the blades is variable as it has a sliding lock. The lock is sliding type with a claw handle and a fish tail end. The advantage of the sliding lock is that it can deliver the head by asynclitism. It is a long heavy forceps and is associated with severe maternal injuries.

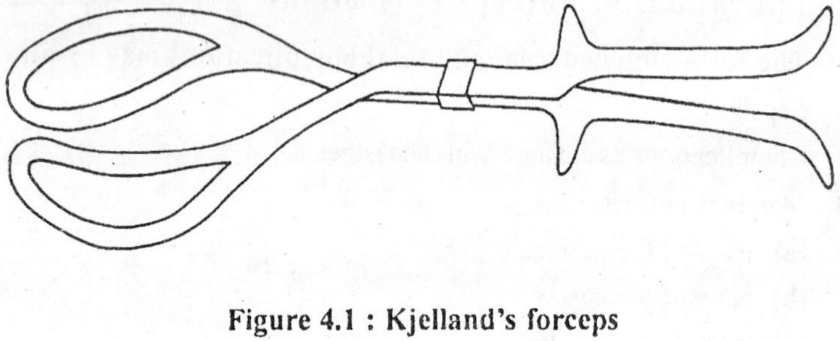

Figure 4.1 : Kjelland's forceps

Uses

1. This forceps is now obsolete. It was earlier used for high forceps operations with the biparietal diameter lying above the pelvic brim but now this operation has been discarded. The methods used, i.e. direct, indirect and classical have already been described in this text.

2. It can be used for rotation and extraction of head in persistent occipitoposterior positions or deep transverse arrest. The absence of a well defined pelvic curve makes it a useful instrument for rotating the head.

HAIGH FERGUSON'S FORCEPS WITH AXIS TRACTION ROD

It is a midcavity forceps which can be used with or without the axis traction apparatus. It has both cephalic and pelvic curves, the maximum distance between the closed blades being 3 inches and between tips being 3 cm. The lock is fixed French type. The forceps is 13.5 inches long with slots in the blades. The blades are known as the application handles and have a fish tail appearance. The axis traction rod is a the single traction handle which fits into the application handles. It consists of a transverse bar with slots for the shanks and a ball and socket joint. The fenestration or slots in the blades were earlier used for threading tape into them in order to apply traction. The Pajot's manoeuvre can be used in place of the axis traction apparatus. The advantage of the axis traction rod with a ball and socket joint is that the rotation of the head is not hampered as it descends down.

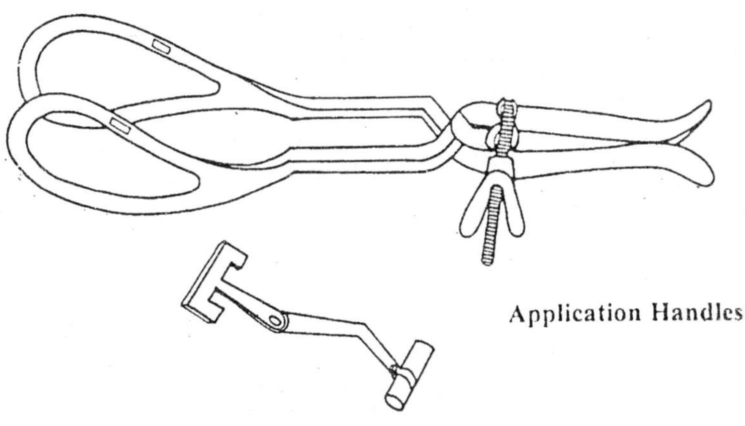

Figure 4.2 : Haigh Ferguson's forceps with axis traction rod

Uses

1. For a midforceps application in a rotated head with or without axis traction.
2. For a mid forceps application with axis traction to unrotated head.
3. For an outlet forceps delivery without axis traction.

WRIGLEY'S SHORT CURVED OBSTETRIC FORCEPS

It is a small light forceps about one third the weight of a long obstetric forceps. The length is only 11 inches and this reduction is achieved by reducing the size of the shanks of the forceps and its handles. The maximum distance between closed blades is 3 inches and between tips is 1 inch. It has a English type fixed lock.

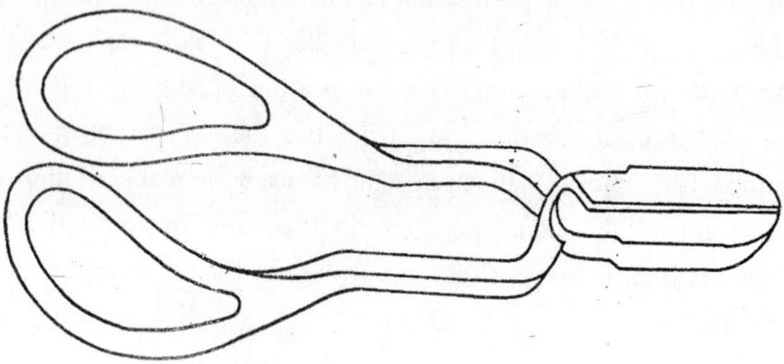

Figure 4.3 : Wrigley's short curved obstetric forceps

Uses

It is used as an outlet forceps when the head is at or below +2 station.

VENTOUSE OR VACUUM EXTRACTOR

It is a device which delivers the baby by gentle traction on its head. The instrument consists of a cup which is made to adhere to the fetal head by means of vacuum, i.e. negative pressure is created. The apparatus consists of :

1. Ball shaped steel suction cups or silastic cups of 40 mm, 50 mm and 60 mm size.
2. A traction chain, covered by rubber tubing.
3. A traction bar.
4. A suction tubing made of rubber connecting the traction bar to the suction apparatus which creates a negative pressure by removing air or a separate opening for attachment of suction tubing.
5. A manometer which is connected to the suction apparatus for pressure recordings.

Technique

The perineum is locally infiltrated with xylocaine or a pudendal block is given with full aseptic precautions. Bladder and bowel should be emptied. The appropriate sized cup is chosen and applied to the fetal scalp after making sure that the cervix or the vagina are not included. The rubber tubing is attached to the suction pump and a pressure of 0.2 atmospheres is created. An artificial caput succedaneum is formed after several minutes and pressure is now increased to 0.4 and then 0.6 atmospheres taking atleast 20 minutes for it. The caput so formed is known as the 'Chignon'. The traction applied should be intermittent and with the uterine contractions. The direction of pull should be at right angles to the surface to which the cup is applied. As the head descends down, episiotomy is applied and when the head is delivered the cup is removed gently off the 'Chignon'.

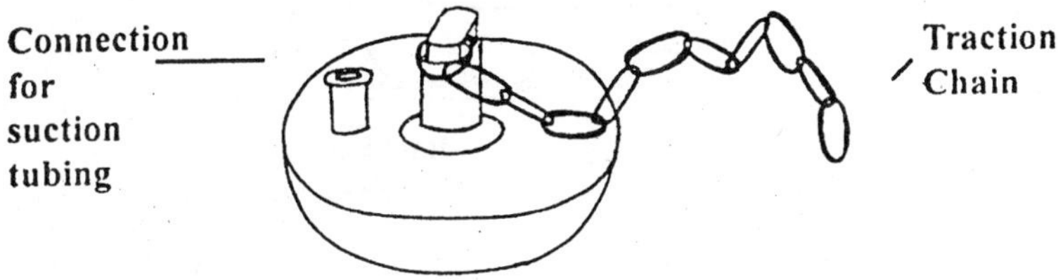

Figure 4.4 : Ventouse suction cup

Uses

1. It is an alternative to the obstetric forceps in the second stage of labour with the cervix fully dilated and the head low in the pelvis.
2. In the first stage of labour, it can be of help as soon as the cervix is dilated enough to allow safe application of the cups in case of ineffective uterine contractions or malrotation.
3. It can be used along with symphysiotomy in mild to moderate cases of disproportion.

Complications and disadvantages

1. Injury to maternal tissues but rare as compared to obstetric forceps.
2. Cannot help in case of fetal distress unlike the obstetric forceps as it needs time for chignon to form.
3. Cephalhematoma, intracranial injuries and necrosis of fetal scalp may result.
4. Can be used only in vertex positions.
5. Cannot be used in premature babies.

Advantages over obstetric forceps

1. Less traumatic than the obstetric forceps.
2. Does not require space in a cramped pelvis.
3. Can be applied even to a cervix which is not fully dilated.
4. Can be applied to an unrotated head as its rotates the head with descent.

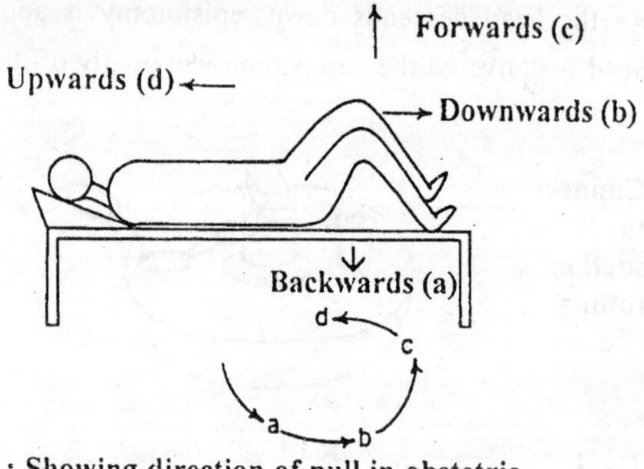

Figure 4.5 : Showing direction of pull in obstetric forceps and ventouse

Chapter V

Instruments used for Destructive Operations

These instruments are designed to reduce the bulk of the fetal head or trunk in order to facilitate its delivery through the vagina. The liberal use and increasing safety of the caesarean section has limited the use of these operations but they still have a role to play in the developing and the underdeveloped countries. The following operations are used :

I. **Craniotomy :** It includes.

1. Perforation of the head and drainage of CSF and brain matter.
2. Extraction of the perforated head by.
   (a) Slow expulsive maternal efforts.
   (b) Extraction with obstetric forceps but may slip off causing maternal injuries.
   (c) Extraction with Braxton Hicks–2–bladed cranioclast by crushing of the cranium.
   (d) Extraction after crushing by Winter's 3-bladed cephalotribe, i.e., cephalotripsy.
   (e) Cranioclasm or extraction after crushing and avulsion of cranial vault and crushing the base of the skull & face.

II. **Decapitation of the head.**

III. **Evisceration**

IV. **Cliedotomy**

V. **Pubiotomy and Symphysiotomy.**

The following instruments are used in craniotomy.

(b) after coming head of breech

(c) face presentation with obstructed labour

(d) failed forceps operation due to cephalopelvic disproportion.

The parietal bones in case of the forecoming head, the occipital bone in aftercoming head and the orbits in brow presentation are the sites for perforation. Perforation is done only during a uterine contraction after fixing the presenting part from above. The blades of the perforator are closed and fixed and introduced after protecting the maternal tissues with a hand such that palms face the blades. Full asepsis is maintained. The blades are guided to the skull by the right hand while left hand protects the maternal tissues. An assistant fixes the head suprapubically and the perforator is pushed in till the level of the shoulder. It is then opened up and rotated by 90° after closing the blades. After rotation, the blades are again opened up and a cruciate incision is thus obtained and brain matter is crushed with it. Suprapubic pressure will now drain out the brain matter or it may be drained by the help of a flushing curette or suction canula or a Drewsmythes catheter.

Complications

Severe maternal lacerations and even uterine rupture may result.

DREW SMYTHE'S CATHETER

It is a long double curved instrument, sinusoidal in shape with a double opening. There is an inlet and an outlet and a double tube.

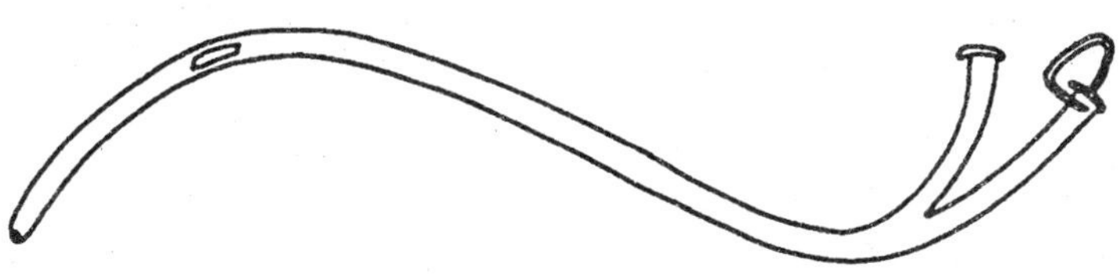

Figure 5.2 : Drew smythe's catheter

Uses

1. High rupture of membranes as in hydramnios to prevent cord prolapse and accidental hemorrhage due to sudden decompression.
2. For perforation of a hydrocephalic aftercoming head of breech through the foramen magnum or a spina bifida or by dividing the vertebral canal in the cervical region.
3. For draining a forecoming hydrocephalic head after perforating it with scissors.

CHURCHILL'S BONE NIBBLER

It is a curved forceps with a handle and a lock. The blades have strong serrations for crushing any bony spicules after perforation to prevent trauma to the birth canal during extraction of the head.

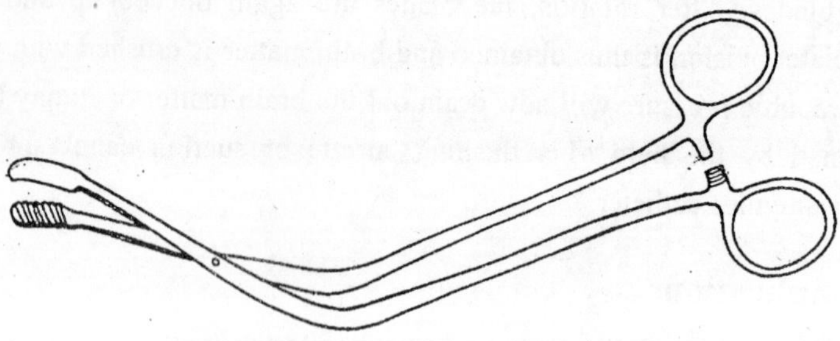

Figure 5.3 : Churchill's bone nibbler

FLUSHING CURETTE

It is a metallic spoon shaped canula used to remove brain matter by flushing it out after attaching it to an enema can with a rubber tubing.

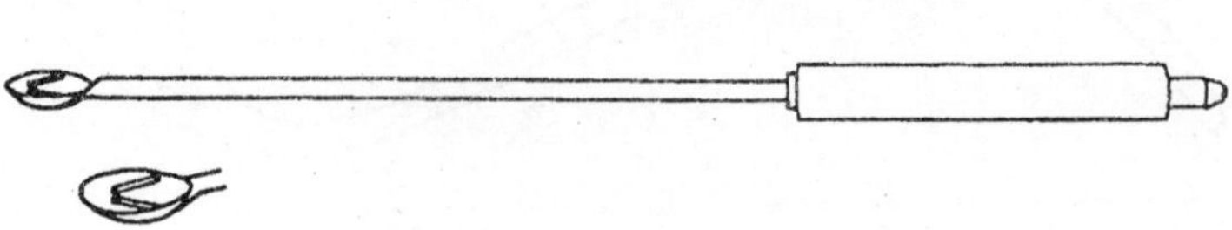

Figure 5.4 : Flushing curette

TWO-BLADED BRAXTON HICKS'S CRANIOCLAST

It consists of the central and the left outer blade of the Winter's cephalotribe. The smaller solid central blade is pointed and acts as a perforator while the large curved fenestrated outer blade acts as a crusher. The opposed surfaces of the blades are strongly serrated and the handles are firmly closed by a screw and locked. The pointed central blade perforates the skull and is screwed into the foramen magnum while the outer blade is placed outside between the scalp and the bones. The firm grip on the head and some amount of crushing action helps by negotiating cephalopelvic disproportion. It can also be used for the avulsion of the bones of the vault, i.e., cranioclasm operation.

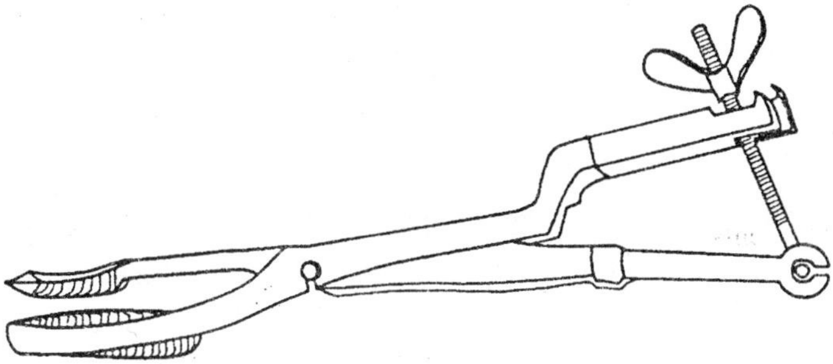

Figure 5.5 : Two-bladed Braxton Hicks's cranioclast

WINTER'S 3-BLADED CEPHALOTRIBE

It is used for extraction of a perforated head after crushing it. The middle blade is screwed into the foramen magnum through the perforation aperture and is held by an assistant. The first outer blade is passed over the face and then screwed up with the central blade to crush the face. The second outer blade is then passed up over the occiput and screwed up with the central blade. If properly applied the reduction in the size of the skull is considerable and a firm grip is obtained for extraction. But before extraction the perforation aperture must be examined for the presence of any bony spicules to avoid maternal injuries. The direction of pull is along the axis of the pelvis.

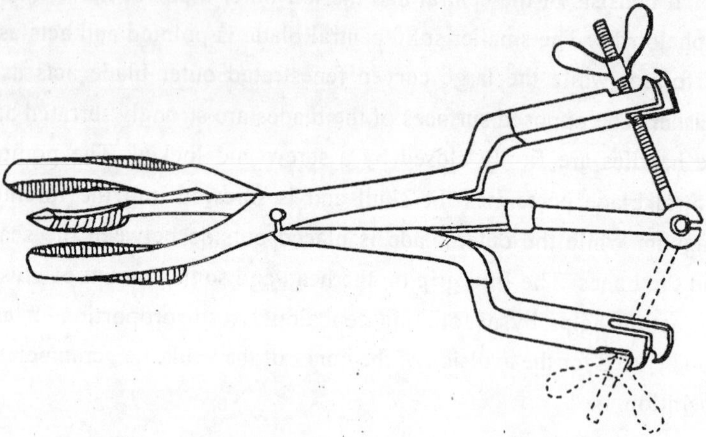

Figure 5.6 : Winter's 3-bladed cephalotribe

WILLET'S SCALP TRACTION FORCEPS

This forceps has 2 blades shaped like the letter 'T' and a handle with a lock. The blades have oblique serrations on the inner aspect and one of the blades has 2 small spikes which fit into corresponding holes on the other blade:

The spikes, transverse serrations and the lock provide a firm grip of the fetal scalp. The instrument has no role in modern obstetrics except when the baby is dead.

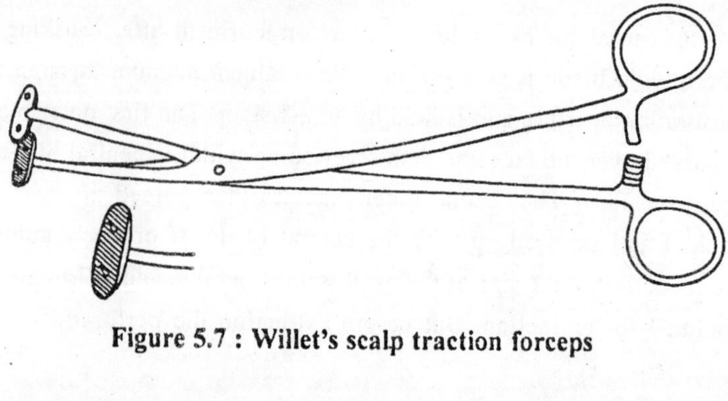

Figure 5.7 : Willet's scalp traction forceps

Uses

1. It is used in cases of placenta previa when the patient is bleeding profusely and facilities for cesarean section are not available. To save the life of the mother a quick rupture of the membranes is done and the fetal head is pulled down with the forceps. A small weight is applied to it for traction. The bleeding is controlled by the compression of the placental bed from the pressure exerted by the fetal head.
2. To extract the fetal head after perforation during a craniotomy operation.
3 To hasten the delivery of an old IUD baby with a collapsed head which is unable to act as a good dilator for the cervix.

Complications

1. Lacerations and avulsion of the fetal scalp.
2. Haemorrhage from fetal scalp injury.
3. Fetal scalp infection.
4. Accidental injury to maternal tissues

DECAPITATION

In this operation the head of the baby is severed from the neck and the two parts are delivered per vaginum. The indications are:

1. Transverse lie with impacted shoulder.
2. Locked twins
3. Conjoined twins
4. Double-headed monster.

The following instruments are used in decapitation.

RAMSBOTHAM'S DECAPITATION SAW

It has a blade, shaped like a wide hook with a bent tip and a serrated inner edge. The other end has a transverse bar serving as a handle.

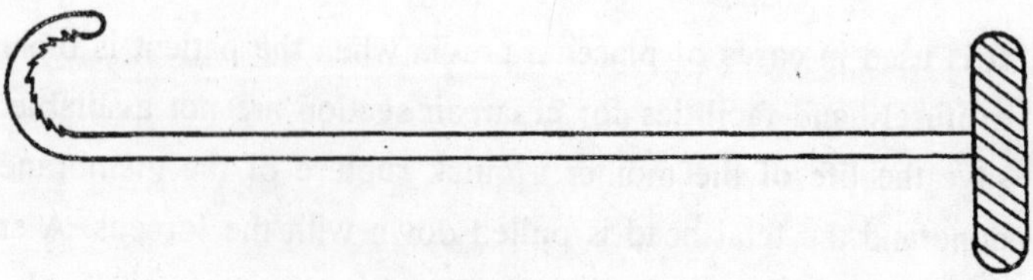

Figure 5.8 : Ramsbotham's decapitation saw

The prolapsed hand in a transverse lie is pulled down or if not already prolapsed then it is made to prolapse. The saw is introduced under cover of the palmar surface of the left hand keeping the tip towards the occiput. When the neck of the baby is reached the saw is rotated by 90° to guide the cutting edge along the neck of the baby. The decapitation is started by gentle to and fro sawing movements until the bones are severed. The remaining soft tissues of the neck are cut with embryotomy scissors. The baby is delivered by pulling on the arm after checking that no bony spicules are present which can damage maternal tissues or it may be delivered by version. The severed head is delivered by :

1. Putting a finger in the mouth and applying traction.
2. By forceps.
3. By craniotomy
4. By crochet and hook

BRAUN'S DECAPITATION HOOK

It is a blunt instrument with a narrow hook and a bulbous tip. It is passed up in a manner similar to a decapitation saw until the vertebral column in the neck region is reached then suddenly rotated with a jerky movement in order to dislocate the vertebrae. The soft tissues are then cut with scissors. The severed head and the trunk are delivered as after decapitation with the decapitation saw.

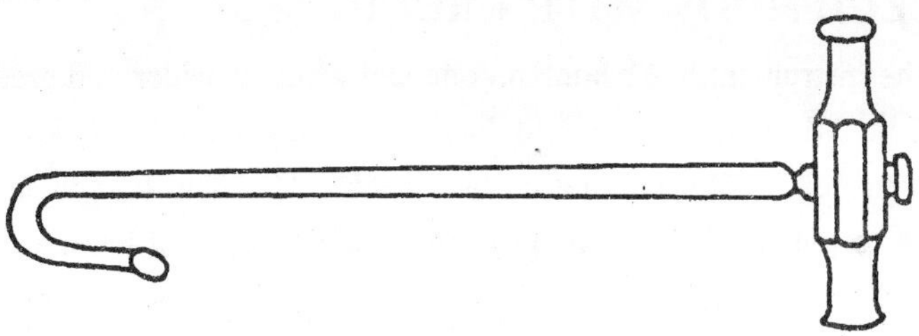

Figure 5.9 : Braun's decapitation hook

BLOND-HIEDLER'S DECAPITATION SAW WIRE WITH THIMBLE

It consists of a thimble with a ring, a 43 cm long wire, saw blade with a rubber sheath at each end and 2 handles. The rubber sheath covers about 1/3 of the length of the wire saw to prevent damage to the surrounding area. Each end has a small metal ball on which traction handles may be fitted. It is a safer and more effective instrument for decapitation. It is supplied with the aid of a metal thimble on the operators thumb which temporarily carries one end of the saw and is made to encircle the neck of the baby. The sawing is then done after applying traction handles.

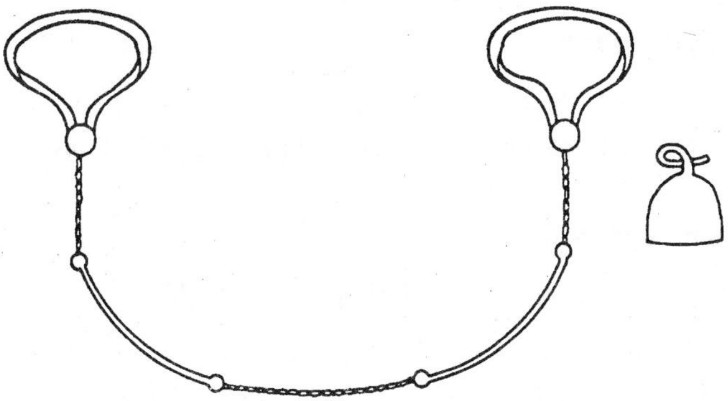

Figure 5.10 : Blond-Hiedler's decapitation saw with thimble

BREECH HOOK WITH CROCHET

The instrument has a hook on one end which is wider and gradually bent while the other end has an acutely bent hook known as the crotchet. The curvatures face each other. The breech hook is used to put traction on the groin in case of impacted breech of a dead fetus. The crotchet part is used to hook down a decapitated head through the mouth or a hole in the skull.

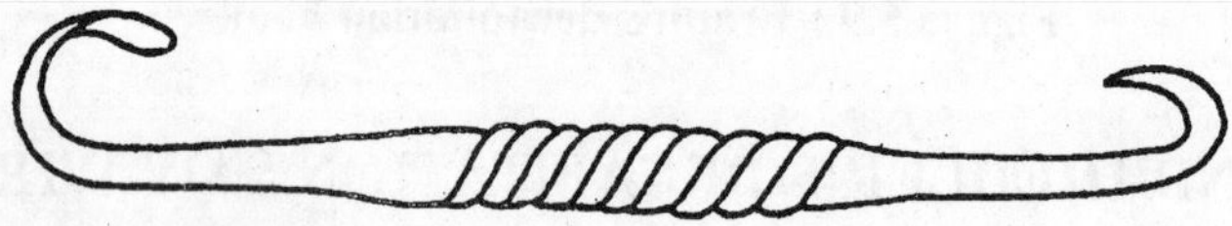

Figure 5.11 : Breech hook with crochet

EVISCERATION

Here the abdomen or the thorax is opened up by strong scissors and the viscera is removed to debulk and deliver the baby.

Indications

1. Shoulder presentation with dead baby.
2. Fetal ascites.
3. Cystic kidneys of the baby leading to an enlarged abdomen.

CLIEDOTOMY

One or both the clavicles are divided with a strong pair of scissors only in case of a dead fetus in the following indications:

1. Large baby
2. Narrow pelvic outlet.

PUBIOTOMY AND SYMPHYSIOTOMY

Pubiotomy involves the divisi‹ n of the body of the pubes while symphysiotomy involves divisio· of the symphysis pubis joint. They help by increasing the diametr of the pelvis for the delivery of the baby.

Chapter VI

Instruments used for Operations on Ovarian Cysts

SPENCER WELL'S TROCAR AND CANULA

It consists of a hollow outer tube and a sharply pointed trocar which projects beyond the hollow outer canula. The trocar is introduced into the ovarian cyst for puncturing it and the outer tube is firmly fixed to the surface. The trocar is now withdrawn and the cyst fluid is sucked out until the cyst collapses to the required size. The cyst which is now reduced in size can be removed after closing the puncture site with a Pyesmith's forceps clip to prevent spillage and dissemination into the peritoneal cavity.

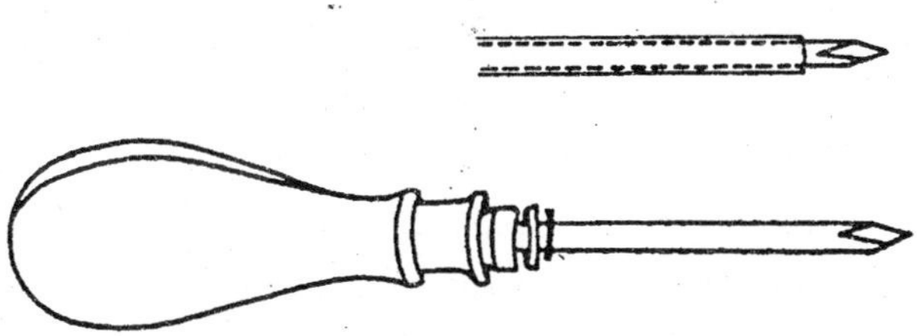

Figure 6.1 : Spencer Well's trocar and canula

Uses

1. For draining huge ovarian cysts to facilitate their easy removal.
2. To drain the CSF from a hydrocephalic baby and deliver it vaginally.

PYESMITH'S FORCEPS CLIP

It is a forceps with blades designed like a 'question mark' and having serrations on the inner side, a lock and finger grips. The forceps is used to close the puncture site of an ovarian cyst when the trocar and canula are withdrawn after draining the cyst. It prevents spillage of cyst fluid into the peritoneal cavity and prevents its dissemination into the peritoneal cavity.

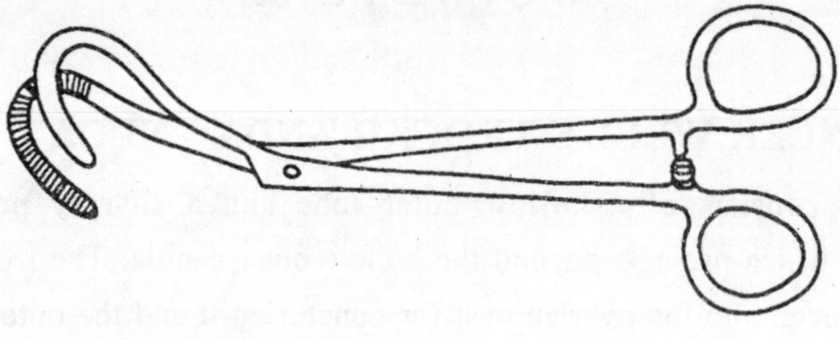

Figure 6.2 : Pyesmith's forceps clip

NELATON'S CYST HOLDING FORCEPS

The instrument consists of two blades, a lock and a handle with finger grips. The blades are rounded with a central fenestration and transverse serrations on the inner aspect. There are four spikes on one blade which fit into corresponding holes on the other blade. The instrument is used to hold a cyst before identifying its pedicle. Though the spikes give an excellent grip of the cyst it cannot be used to hold a tense cyst. Also, it can cause rupture of the cyst. The instrument is not used now and has become obsolete.

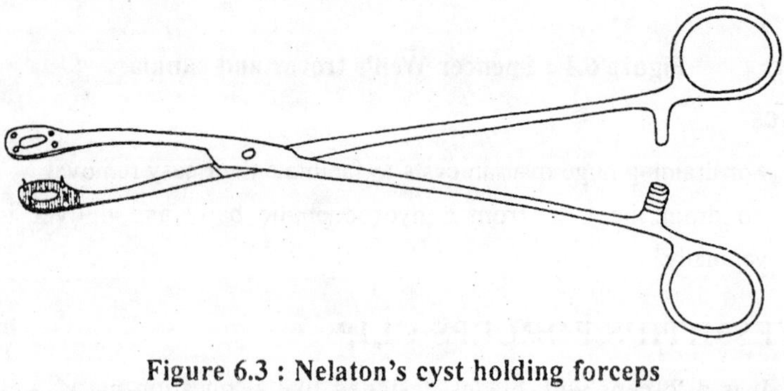

Figure 6.3 : Nelaton's cyst holding forceps

Chapter VII

Specialised Gynaecological Instruments

UTERINE POLYP FORCEPS

It is used for the removal of endometrial polyps. It has slender blades ending in flattened ovals. The blades have fenestrations and transverse serrations. The instrument has a joint, handles with finger grips and a lock for a firm grip of the polyp.

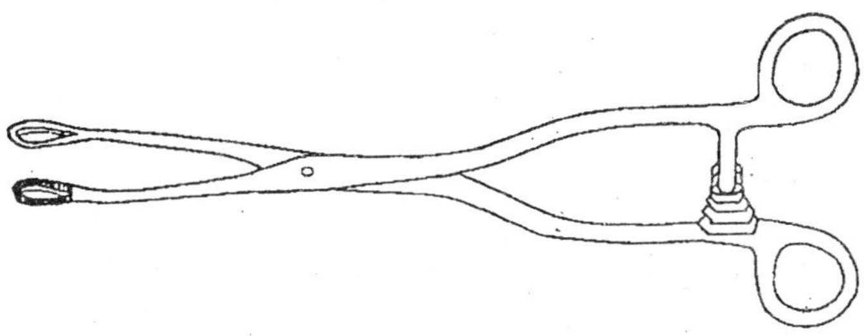

Figure 7.1 : Uterine polyp forceps

Technique

After full asepsis and retraction of anterior and posterior vaginal walls the cervix is grasped with a volsellum. The polyp holding forceps is introduced into the uterine cavity after dilatation of cervical canal. The forceps is locked after getting a firm hold of the polyp, and the polyp is removed by twisting resulting in its avulsion. A check curettage is done and if the bleeding is excessive then the cavity may be packed for sometime.

Uses

This forceps is used for the removal of :

1. Uterine mucus polyp.
2. Uterine myomatous polyp
3. Uterine placental polyp.
4. Cervical polyps, both adenomatous and fibroid type.

Uterine Dressing forceps

It is a long, straight instrument with a lock and transverse serrations on the inner aspect. It is used to swab the uterine cavity.

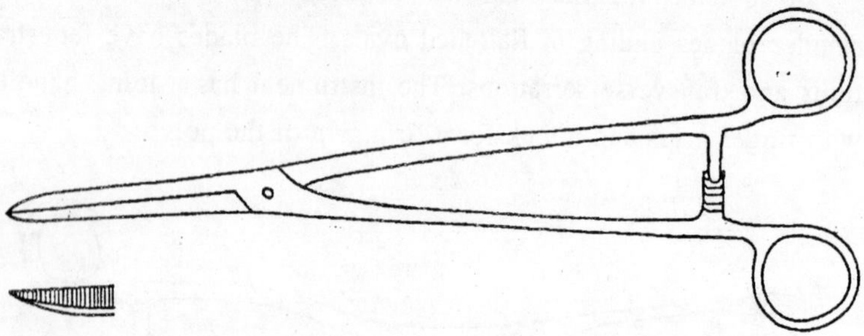

Figure 7.2 : Uterine dressing forceps

Technique

A small piece of gauze is held between the blades and introduced inside the uterine cavity and all the walls and the fundal area of the uterus are cleaned by gently rotating it all around.

Uses

To swab the uterine cavity after :

1. Suction and evacuation
2. Draining of pyometra
3. Draining of haematometra

Disadvantages

1. Injury may occur in the vagina, uterus or cervix.

2. A small piece of swab or threads may be left behind and may serve as nidus for infection.

Uterus packing forceps

It is a long, slender sinuously curved instrument having blades and handles. The blades have transverse serrations on the inside so a firm grip is obtained. It is used to pack the uterine cavity in cases of PPH to control bleeding.

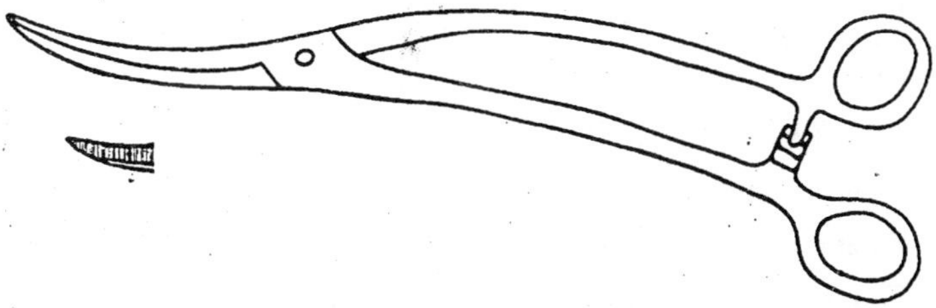

Figure 7.3 : Uterus packing forceps

Technique

A check curettage is done to rule out retained placental bits as a cause of postpartum hemorrhage. The cervix is grasped with a sponge holder after retracting the vaginal walls. A sterilised ribbon gauze is introduced and packing is started from one cornual end to the other and back again till the whole cavity is packed. The cervix and vagina should also be packed alongwith uterine packing. If one ribbon gauze is insufficient another maybe attached to it with a firm knot and the number of ribbons used should be noted down. Care should be taken not to leave any dead space at the fundus or in between as bleeding will occur and defeat the purpose of packing. The patient is watched carefully for any deterioration of vitals, bleeding per vaginum or increase in fundal height. These events suggest continuing uterine bleed and failure of the procedure and decision for hysterectomy or internal iliac artery ligation be taken immediately.

Uses

I. It is used for uterine packing in :

1. Uncontrolled atonic post-partum hemorrhage.
2. Uncontrolled post abortal hemorrhage.
3. Bleeding from the uterus after polypectomy, not controlled by curettage.

II. For vaginal packing:

1. After vaginal hysterectomy to control oozing from vault.
2. After cervical or vaginal biopsy.
3. To control oozing from a ragged cervix after delivery.
4. To control secondary hemorrhage after operations like vaginal hysterectomy, fothergill's repair, conisation, etc.
5. After insertion of laminaria tents or intrauterine radium needles to prevent their expulsion.

Disadvantages

The following complications may occur :

1. Intrauterine collection of blood may be missed unless fundal height is carefully monitored.
2. Sepsis
3. Injury by the instrument.
4. Asherman's syndrome specially if sepsis occurs.
5. Placental anomalies like placenta accreta in subsequent pregnancies.
6. Procedure may fail and patient may require a major operation with precious time being lost in between.

Advantages

1. It is a useful measure to control postpartum hemorrhage specially in cases where the patient has not completed her family and wants to conserve her reproductive capability.
2. It also helps in avoiding major operations like a hysterectomy in a patient with poor general condition.

IUCD REMOVING HOOK

It is a long, angled instrument resembling a uterine sound with the difference that it is not graduated and has hooks at the distal end subterminally.

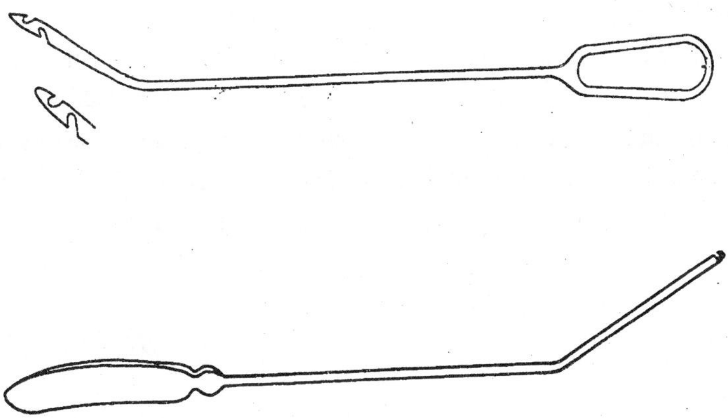

Figure 7.4 : IUCD removing hooks

Technique

It is an out patient operation which does not require anaesthesia or cervical dilatation. The hook is passed inside the uterine cavity with full asepsis and after exposing the cervix. The IUCD is hooked out and it is checked that IUCD has been completely removed with no broken ends remaining inside.

Uses

1. Removal of IUCD when the threads at the tail end have rolled up and are missing.
2. Removal of a tubal prosthesis per vaginum.

Disadvantages

1. Can cause cervical injuries or perforation of uterus.
2. Can damage the endometrium by repeated attempts to remove the IUCD.

CERVICAL PUNCH BIOPSY FORCEPS

It is a strong stout instrument with 2 blades, handles with finger grips and a lock. The blades consist of one smaller blade with a sharp cutting edge that fits closely into the larger blade which holds the specimen like a basket. The handles are angulated to avoid obstruction of the field of vision while taking the biopsy.

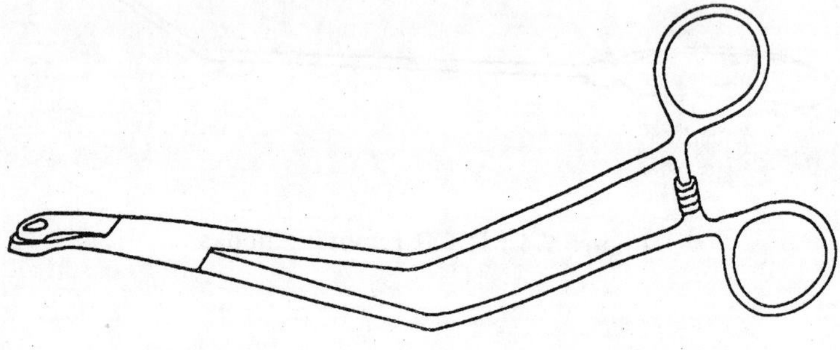

Figure 7.5 : Cervical punch biopsy forceps

Technique

Operation does not require any anaesthesia or sedation. Para cervical block may be given. Full aseptic precautions are taken. The site of biopsy should be such that both the abnormal area and a part of normal area are included in the specimen for a proper comparison. The suspicious area can be demarcated by painting with Schiller's iodine or by a colpomicroscope. The raw area after biopsy may bleed and haemostasis can be done by taking one or two stitches or by packing the vagina. The tissue is sent for HPE in formalin vials.

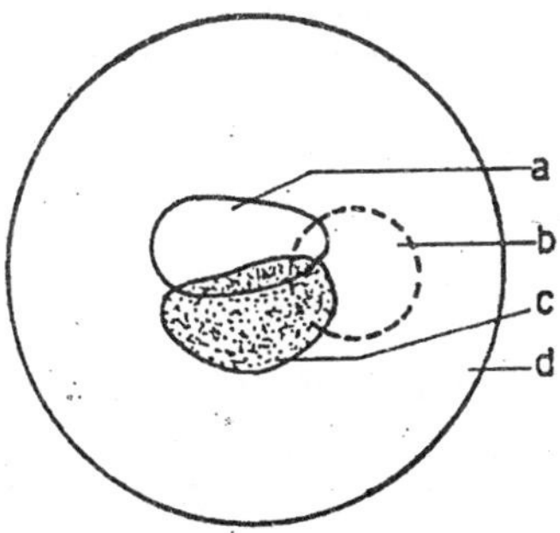

Figure 7.6 : Showing method of taking punch biopsy (a) External os, (b) Punch biopsy site, (c) Cervical lesion and (d) Cervix

Uses

1. Recurrent cervicitis with non healing erosions not responding to antibiotics, i.e., 'bad cervix'.
2. Post coital bleeding.
3. Abnormal Pap's smears.
4. Non-healing ulcers on the cervix.
5. Abnormal finding on Schiller's test or colpomicroscopy.

Disadvantages

The following complications can occur :

1. Sepsis
2. Hemorrhage.

DOYEN'S RING HANDLE MYOMA SCREW

It consists of a cockscrew like arrangement ending in a pointed tip and a handle.

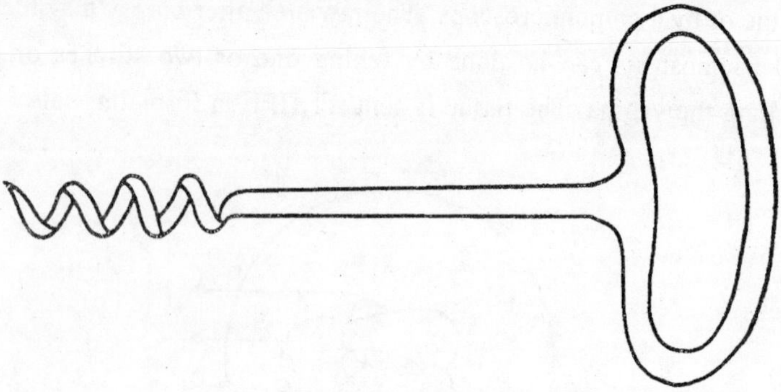

Figure 7.7 : Doyen's myoma screw

Uses

1. The instrument is used to stabilise or fix a myoma during myomectomy after incising its capsule.
2. It can also be used to steady a bulky uterus during hysterectomy.

BONNEY'S MYOMECTOMY CLAMP

The instrument consists of blades at an angle of 120° to the shaft, a joint and handles with a lock. The blades have an overlapping transverse bar dividing it into two compartments. The anterior half of this compartment is covered by rubber tubing which prevents trauma to the structures held. The handles have 2 pairs of finger grips, a proximal and a distal one. The instrument is used during certain operations on the uterus to reduce intra operative blood loss.

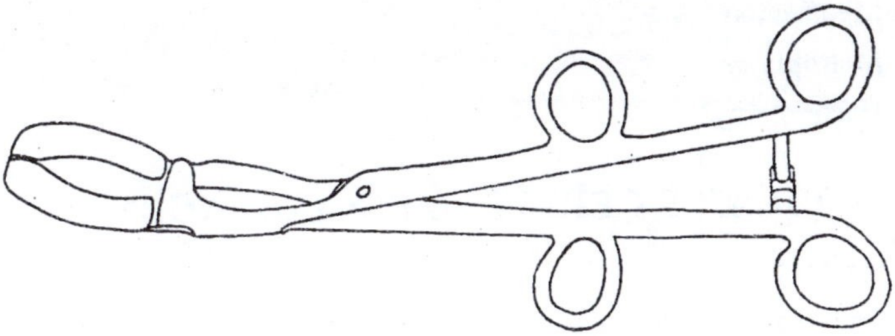

Figure 7.8 : Bonney's myomectomy clamp

Technique

The instrument is applied with its curve downwards, facing the symphysis pubis. In cases of fibroid it can be applied with the curve upwards if the distorted shape of the uterus so requires. The distal finger grips are used for applying and removing the instrument. The proximal finger grip is used for application of the instrument when uterus is much enlarged, as it can open up the instrument to a wider extent with a greater degree of mechanical advantage. The two round ligaments are included in the grip of the blades to prevent the instrument from slipping and to maintain an anteverted position of the uterus. The instrument is applied for clamping the uterine arteries at the level of the internal os. The ovarian artery blood supply is controlled by applying a sponge holder to each infundibulopelvic ligament or by applying intestinal clamps. The clamp is released for a period of 10 minutes after every 20 minutes interval to prevent tissue anoxia and accumulation of harmful substances like histamine, etc. These substances can cause hypotension and shock from vasodilatation if suddenly released into the circulation. The clamp is released only after the myoma bed is obliterated. Haemostasis should be confirmed once the clamp is released.

Uses

To control bleeding in following operations:

1. Myomectomy
2. Metroplasty
3. Hysterotomy

SHIRODKAR'S CERVICAL ENCIRCLAGE NEEDLES

These are two 5 cm long, blunt tipped 1/2 circle needles each having an eye near the tip and attached to a handle at the other end. The needles are designed separately for the right and the left sides with opposite curves, i.e., they are mirror images of each other. They are used to pass a non absorbable encircling suture around the cervix at the level of the internal os. The suture operates by disturbing the uterine polarity and prevents the internal os and the adjacent uterine lower segment from being 'taken up'.

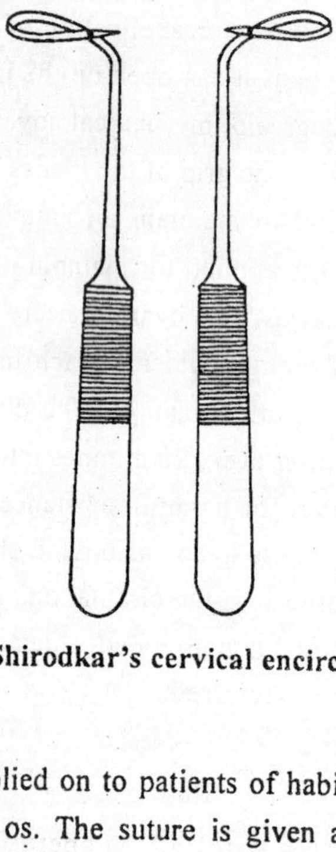

Figure 7.9 : Shirodkar's cervical encirclage needles

Technique

- The suture is applied on to patients of habitual abortion due to incompetent cervical os. The suture is given around 14 weeks of pregnancy or atleast one week before the age of gestation at which the patient usually aborts.

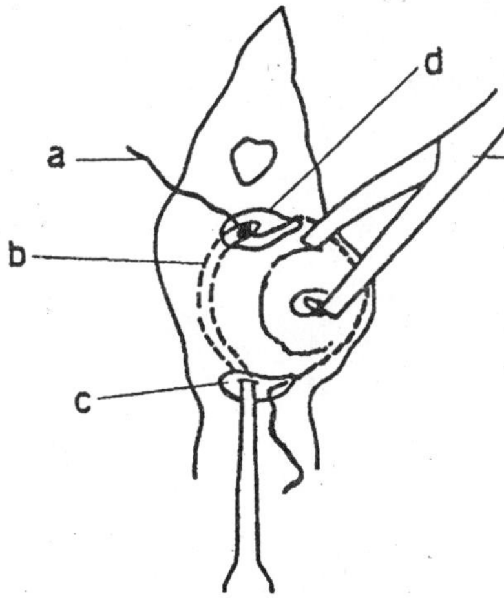

Figure 7.10 : Showing technique of passing encirclage sutures (a) Nonabsorbable suture, (b) Shirodhkar's needle (c) Posterior incision, (d) Anterior incision and (e) Volsellum

The operation is done under general anaesthesia. Full aseptic precautions are taken and a transverse incision is given on the vaginal mucosa at the bladder base. The bladder is pushed up and now another transverse incision is given on the cervico-vaginal junction. The Shirodhkar's needle is introduced beneath the mucosa anteriorly and is made to emerge out posteriorly. A suture is then threaded into the needle and pulled under the mucosa. The steps are similarly repeated on the other side by a mirror image Shirodhkar's needle. The knot can be tied anteriorly or posteriorly but it is preferred to be tied posteriorly to avoid its burying into bladder. After tightening the knot a gap of 3–5 mm should be left in the cervical os. Post operative care after encirclage includes bed rest, prophylactic antibiotics, tocolytic drugs and progesterone. The suture is removed around 36 weeks of pregnancy or immediately if membranes rupture or if the patient goes into premature labour.

Contraindications

1. Rupture of membranes
2. Uterine bleeding
3. Uterine contractions
4. Chorioamnionitis
5. Cervical dilatation more than 4 cm.
6. Polyhydramnios
7. Fetal anomaly

Complications

The complications of encirclage operation range from mild to fatal. These include :

1. Hemorrhage
2. Rupture of membranes
3. Severe infections may occur. The incidence of chorioamnionitis ranges from 15–40% in various studies.
4. Cervical dystocia
5. Uterine rupture
6. Vesico-vaginal fistula
7. Fetal death.

Sommer's Uterus Holding Forceps

The instrument consists of curved blades, a lock and a handle. The blades are at an angle to the shaft so that the operative field is not obstructed. The blades are curved with space in between them to accommodate the uterus without compression. The inner surface of blades has transverse serrations so that the instrument does not slip.

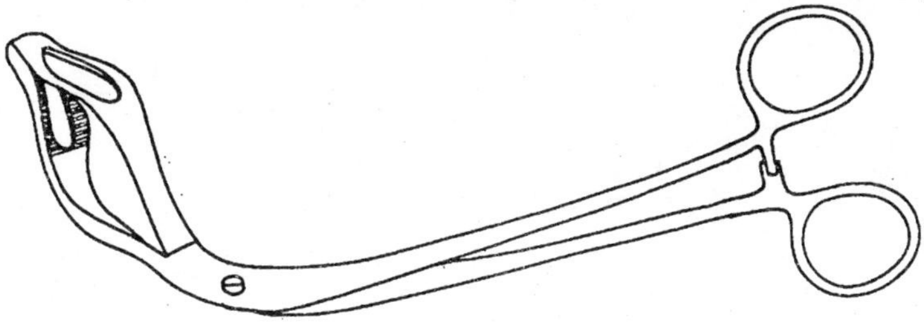

Figure 7.11 : Sommer's uterus holding forceps

Uses

It is used to hold the uterus and to steady it during the following operations :

1. Gilliam's operation for retroversion of the uterus.
2. Tuboplasty operations
3. Salpingostomy, etc. for ectopic pregnancy.
4. VVF and RVF repair by abdominal routes.

Disadvantages

It can not occlude the isthmic region and the cervical canal area. Also, with the instrument in place, any operation on anterior or posterior uterine wall cannot be performed.

Shirodhkar's Uterus Holding Forceps

This instrument has curved blades with distance in between, ending with the transverse bars which are also curved. The transverse bars also have a gap and are covered by rubber tubing to make them atraumatic. These transverse bars occlude the isthmic region and the cervical canal as well. The lock, provides a firm grip and the uterus can be manipulated without slipping.

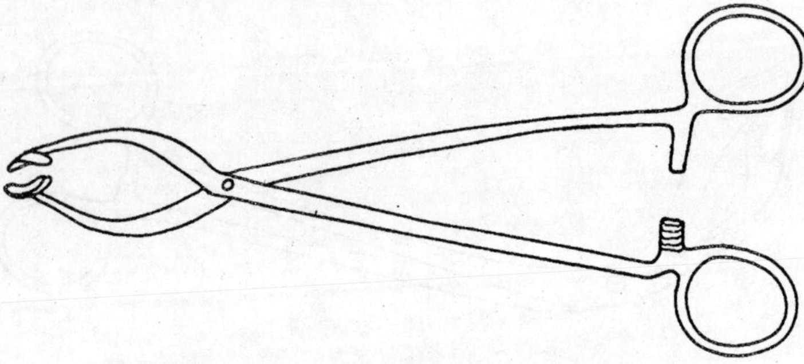

Figure 7.12 : Shirodhkar's uterus holding forceps

Uses

It's uses are similar to those of Sommer's uterus holding forceps.

CAT'S PAW RETRACTOR

It is a long slender instrument with one broader end having a paw-like hook and the other end has a single blunt hook. It was earlier used to bring down abdominal structures during vaginal operations but now has been discarded as it can damage the surrounding structures. The instrument is used in pairs to apply equal traction on both sides of the uterus for pulling it down.

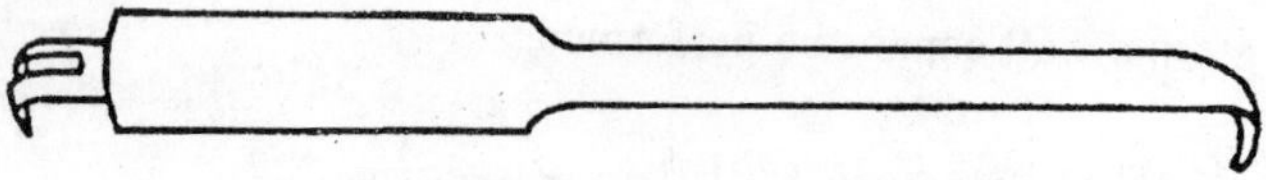

Figure 7.13 : Cat's paw retractor

Uses

1. To bring down the uterus after opening the utero-vesical pouch in vaginal hysterectomy.
2. To bring down the fallopian tubes for vaginal ligations.

LANDON'S BLADDER RETRACTOR

It is a narrow instrument shaped like the letter 'L'. The blade is straight and is at right angles to the handle. The handle is fenestrated for a better grip and to make the instrument lighter.

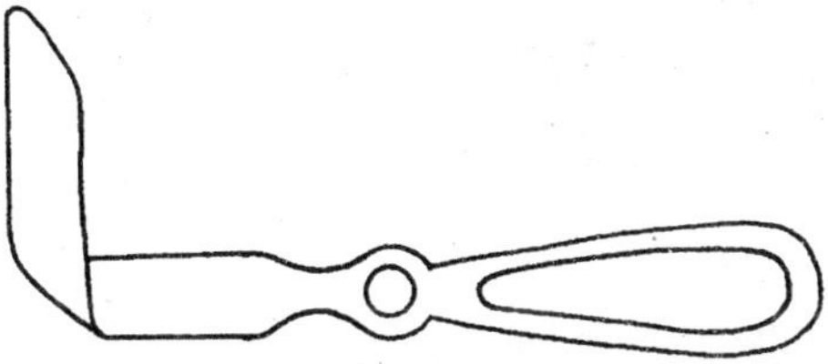

Figure 7.14 : Landon's bladder retractors

Uses

1. To retract the bladder away from the operative field during vaginal hysterectomy after the vesico-vaginal space has been dissected out and bladder has been pushed up.
2. As it is a narrow instrument it can be used for retracting the lateral or anterior vaginal walls during vaginal operations.

GREEN ARMYTAGE CLAMP

The instrument consists of strong, solid triangular blades with transverse serrations, a shaft and a handle with a lock. The flattened broad blades achieve haemostasis over a wider area and can therefore occlude large bleeders.

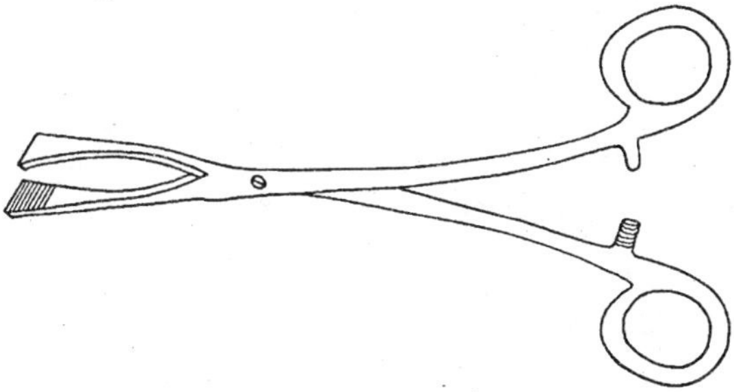

Figure 7.15 : Green Armytage clamp

Uses

1. To hold the cut edges of the uterine scar in cesarean section operation. It helps in compressing the large uterine sinuses and clearly defines the edges for suturing.
2. To hold the angles of the cesarean section scar while suturing.
3. To hold the cervix during its exploration for a cervical tear in place of a sponge holding forceps.

GILLIAM'S NEEDLE

It has a handle a shaft and a curved tip which ends sharply. The tip has an eye for threading.

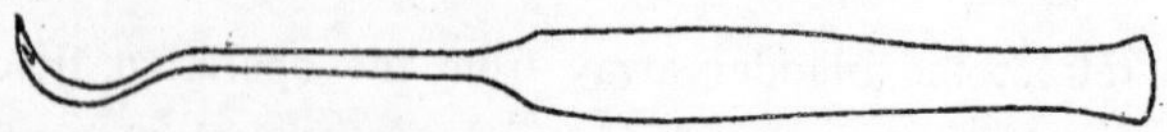

Figure 7.16 : Gilliam's needle

Uses

1. It is used in Gilliam's ventrosuspension operation for a retroverted uterus and ventrosuspension for congenital elongation of cervix along with cervical amputation.
2. It can be used any where when a tubular structure has to be ligated in place of an aneurysm needle.

GLAND DISSECTION FORCEPS

It is a two pronged instrument with blades ending in slightly oval rings. The inner surface of the blades have transverse serrations to provide a firm grip of the structure held. The rounded blades help sin dissection of lymph nodes without causing trauma to the accompanying vessels.

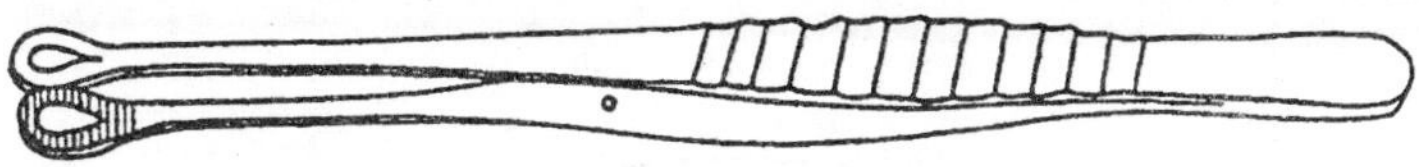

Figure 7.17 : Gland dissection forceps

Uses

The instrument is used for dissecting out lymphnodes during Wertheim's hysterectomy operation.

WERTHEIM'S VAGINAL CLAMP

It is a L–shaped instrument with oblique serrations both in the vertical and horizontal part of the blade. The clamp has a lock and a handle with finger grips. The clamp is applied on the vagina during Wertheim's hysterectomy after the uterus has been separated from its attachments and the cardinal and utero-sacral ligaments have been divided.

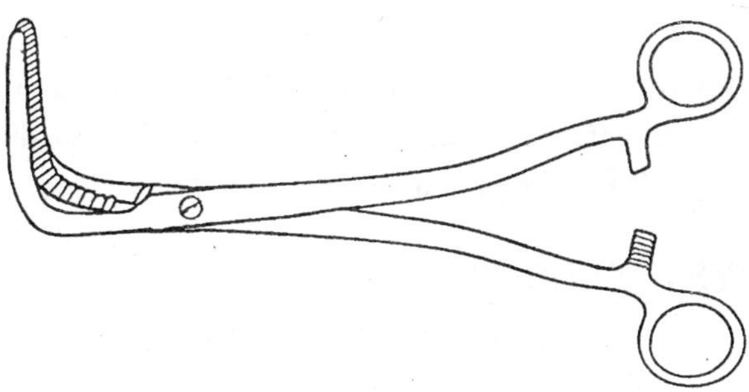

Figure 7.18 : Wertheim's vaginal clamp

It should be applied such that the angle of the clamp lies at the lateral angle of the vagina. The presence of oblique serrations prevents the instrument from slipping while the absence of teeth prevents any trauma to this highly vascular area. The vagina is then cut below the clamp to deliver out the uterus.

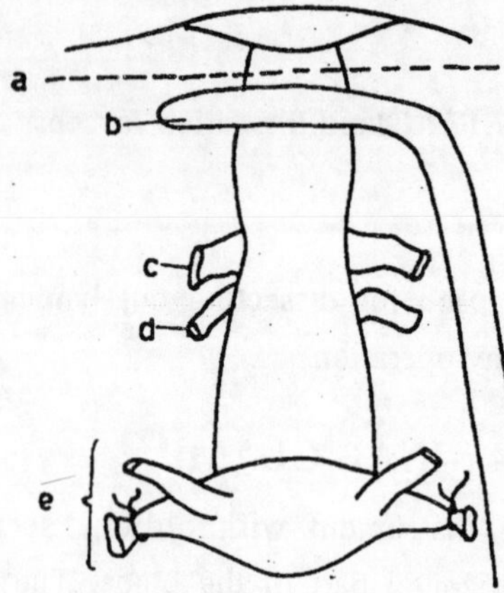

Figure 7.19 : Application of Wertheim's clamp (a) Vaginal cuff, (b) Wertheim's clamp, (c) Mackenrodt's ligament, (d) Uterine artery & (e) Round ligament and infundibulopelvic ligament

Uses

During Wertheim's hysterectomy to prevent the spillage of malignant cells and infective material from the growth onto the raw areas in the pelvis resulting in further spread of the carcinoma.

ANEURYSM NEEDLE

It consists of a rounded needle, a shaft and a handle. The needle has a grooved blunt tip with an eye for threading. It is used to pass a thread around a tubular structure for the application of ligature. The blunt tip cannot penetrate tissues easily so the surrounding structures and vessels are protected from injury. The curved tip gives a mechanical advantage while the grooved eye helps in easy threading of the needle.

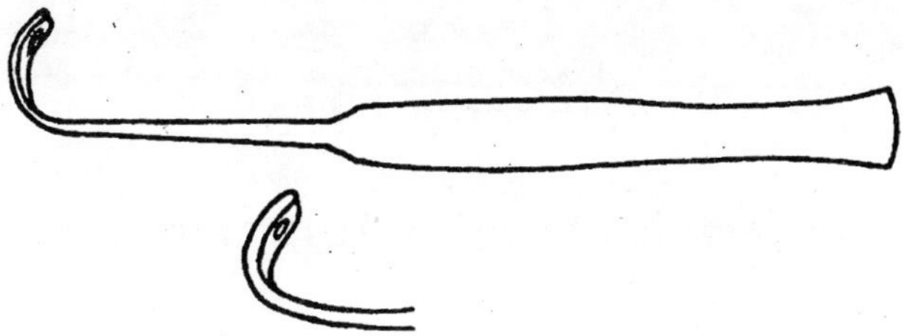

Figure 7.20 : Aneurysm needle

Uses

1. For ligating a vessel around its sheath, e.g. internal iliac ligation for of APH, PPH, etc.
2. Tying a vessel for an aneurysm.
3. During venesection it can be used to ligate a vein.
4. During cut-open operation for starting an IV line.
5. It may be used to ligate pedicles, e.g. renal pedicle, etc.

Chapter VIII

Common Surgical Instruments

KOCHER'S HAEMOSTATIC CLAMP

A long and strong instrument consisting of two blades, a joint, a lock and handle with finger grips. The blades are specially designed to serve the function of efficient haemostats. They have transverse serrations on the inner aspect and are toothed. The transverse serrations, the tooth and the lock together provide a very firm grip of the structure held. It may be of curved type or straight type.

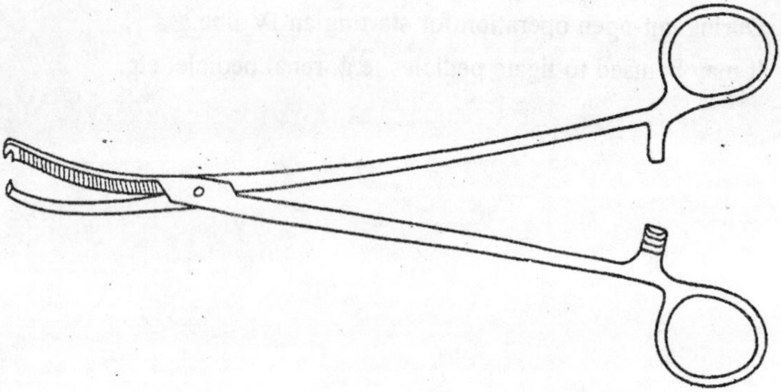

Figure 8.1 : Kocher's haemostatic clamp

Technique

In gynaecological surgery the instrument finds special use in hysterectomy operations for clamping, cutting and ligating the pedicles. Wherever bleeding is expected, the structure is held in between two clamps and then cut and ligated. In exceptionally vascular pedicles with the danger of slipping of ligature double clamps are applied at the pedicle. The ligature is passed and anchored. The assistant first releases the proximal clamp and then the distal one with a slow gentle action while the surgeon tightens the knot.

Uses

1. To clamp, cut and ligate various pedicles like ovarian ligament, Mackenrodts ligament, uterine artery and ovarian artery pedicles in operations like abdominal hysterectomy, vaginal hysterectomy, oophorectomy, salpingectomy, etc.
2. As a clamp for umblical cord.
3. For doing an artificial rupture of membranes in labour.
4. For holding tough structures like rectus sheath while closing the abdomen as in Pfannenstiel incision.

ARTERY FORCEPS

It consists of 2 blades, a joint, a handle with finger grips and a lock. The blades have transverse serrations on the inner aspect. They may be of different types and are named according to the persons who designed them.

1. Small or Halsted mosquito forceps.
2. Medium sized
3. Pedicular type or large artery forceps.

The shape of all above may be straight or curved.

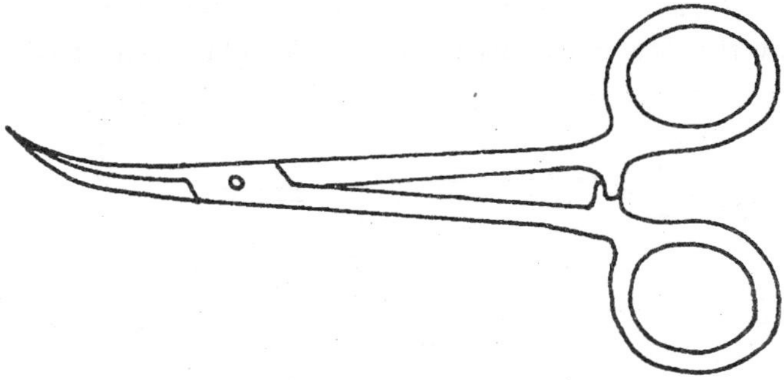

Figure 8.2 : Artery forceps

Technique

Any bleeding point is carefully held between its tips which is then ligated or cauterised by showing the tip to the surgeon.

Uses

1. To hold the bleeders for ligating and cautery.
2. To hold the edges of a wound while suturing it.
3. To hold the free end of a suture.
4. To hold any marker suture (clamped and cut pedicles of Mackenrodts ligament, uterosacral ligaments, etc. in abdominal hysterectomy).
5. To hold retraction sutures for better visibility of the operating field.

NEEDLE HOLDER

It is an instrument used to hold needles while passing sutures during surgery. The shape is similar to an artery forceps but with the difference that the blades are smaller and the serrations on the inner surface are crisscross with a single longitudinal groove to prevent slipping and turning of the needle. The handle has finger bows and a lock for a firm grip.

Types available are :

(a) Straight type also known as Blalock's type.

(b) Curved type also known as Kilner's type. It is used in cavities as the curved handle does not obstruct the view of the operating field.

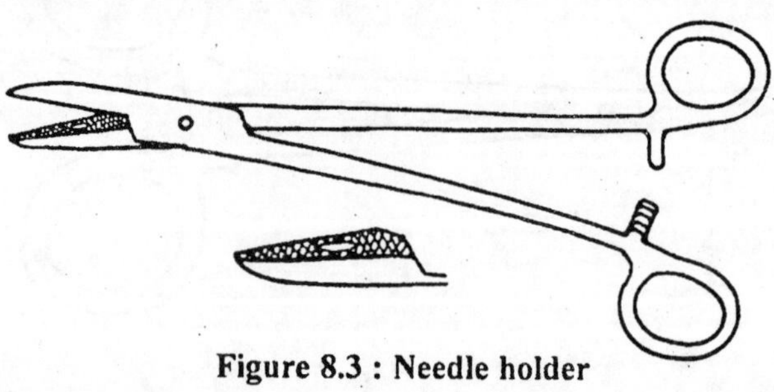

Figure 8.3 : Needle holder

Technique

The needle should be held at the junction of anterior 2/3rd with posterior 1/3rd of its body. If held more posterior the needle may break as this is its weakest points, i.e., near the eye of the needle. If held more towards the middle of the needle there is a mechanical disadvantage and it deforms the shape of the needle.

ALLIS'S TISSUE HOLDING FORCEPS

It is a straight instrument with two blades, and a handle with lock and finger bows. The blades have distance in between and come close together only at the tips and are toothed. The lock and toothed blades provide a firm grip. The teeth are multiple and fine. The space in between the blades prevents trauma and crushing of the structures held. The instrument is available both in a small sizes and large sizes.

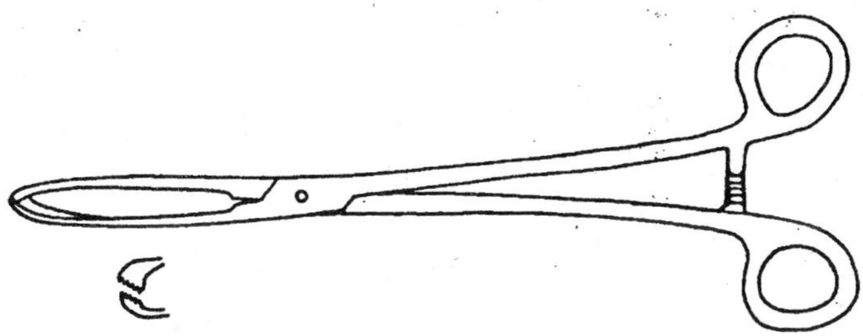

Figure 8.4 : Allis's tissue holding forceps

Uses

1. To hold thin but tough structures like skin and rectus sheath during opening and closure of abdomen.
2. To hold the bleeding edges of the vaginal vault after the uterus has been removed in an abdominal hysterectomy.

3. To hold any fibrous capsule for dissection.
4. To hold the cervix in D & C, HSG, etc.
5. In LSCS for holding the edges of the uterine incision in place of a Green Armytage forceps.
6. To hold the apex of any wound which is being repaired, e.g. episiotomy, perineal tear, etc.
7. As a towel clip.
8. To hold peanut swabs to control oozing in the operation field.

LANES'S TISSUE HOLDING FORCEPS

The blades of this forceps are curved like a spoon, longitudinally fenestrated and the tip is toothed. The handle has a lock. The toothed tip helps in providing a good grip while the fenestrated blade can hold tubular structures without damaging them.

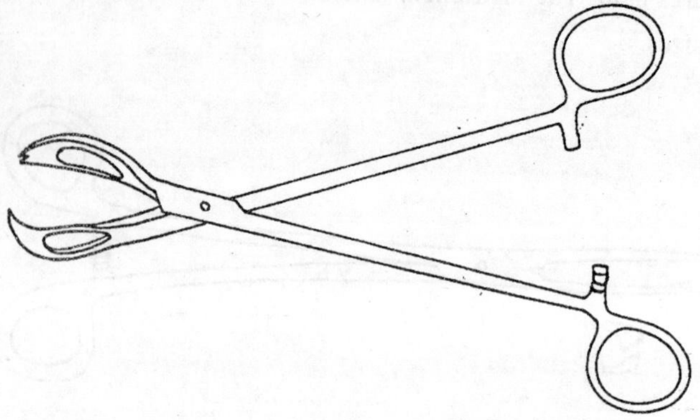

Figure 8.5 : Lanes's tissue holding forceps

Uses

1. To hold thick, tough, structures like rectus sheath lymphnode, lining of a sac, etc.
2. To hold tubular structures like appendix fallopian tubes, ureters, etc., but one has to be careful as the sharp teeth can cause damage.

BABCOCK'S TISSUE HOLDING FORCEPS

It is a light, small instrument with curved fenestrated blades having a transverse bar at the tip. The handles have a lock. The absence of teeth at the tip make it an ideal instrument for holding delicate, soft tubular structures. The fenestrated and curved blades allow the tubular structures to bulge out preventing damage. It comes in 3 sizes; large, medium and small.

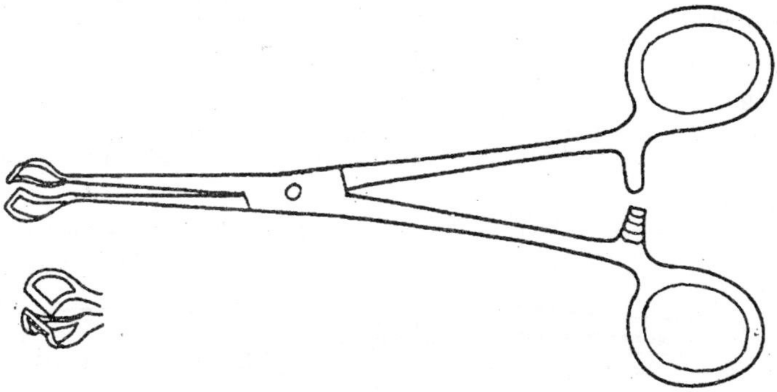

Figure 8.6 : Babcock's tissue holding forceps

Uses

1. To hold the appendix, intestines, spermatic cord, ureters and fallopian tubes, etc.
2. To hold the two levator ani muscles in order to bring them to the centre for approximation in a third degree perineal tear repair operation and posterior colpoperinorrhaphy.
3. To hold bowel, mucosal edges, bladder, etc. in different operation as it causes less trauma.

DISSECTING FORCEPS

These are two-armed instruments used for holding tissues either during dissection or while suturing. They maintain a clear operative field while steadying the part concerned only at the instant required. They can be large or small, fine or heavy and toothed or plain type. They are named after the people who designed them namely Victor's, Lane's, Bonney's and others. The handles have a spring like action and the tips are well apposed and do not slip against each other. The inner aspect of the tips are serrated and outer aspects of the forceps is ridged in the middle for a firm grip on the instrument. The toothed type is used for steadying tough structures while plain type is atraumatic and is used for soft and friable structures like peritoneum.

Uses

Plain type : To hold peritoneum, uterine edges, etc. during suturing.

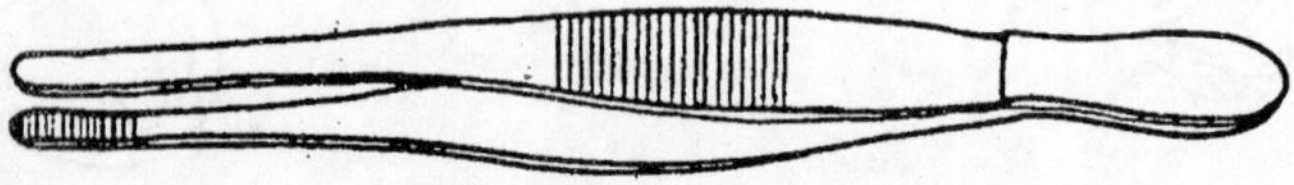

Figure 8.7 : Plain dissecting forceps

Toothed type : To hold tough structures like the edges of vaginal vault, wall, rectus sheath, etc.

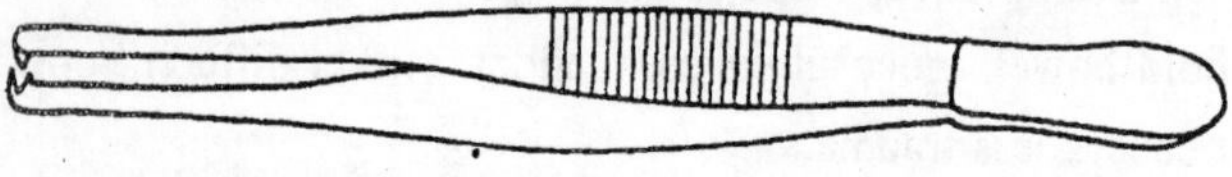

Figure 8.8 : Toothed dissecting forceps

SCISSORS

These are used for blunt as well as sharp dissection and for cutting various pedicles and sutures.

Types

1. Straight scissors :

(a) Blunt

(b) Fine pointed.

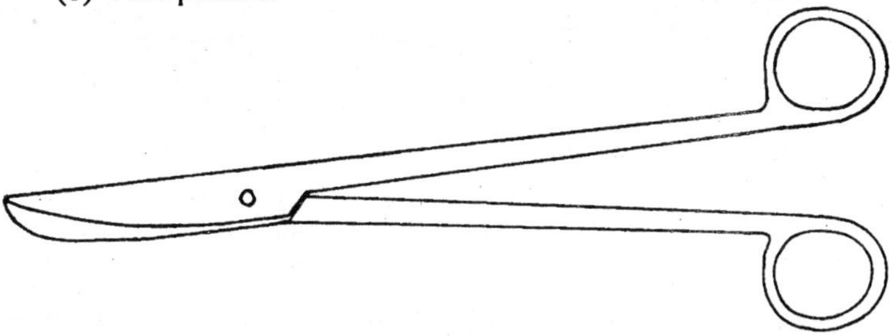

Figure 8.9 : Straight scissors

2. Curved on flat : The curvature at the tip is in the vertical plane.

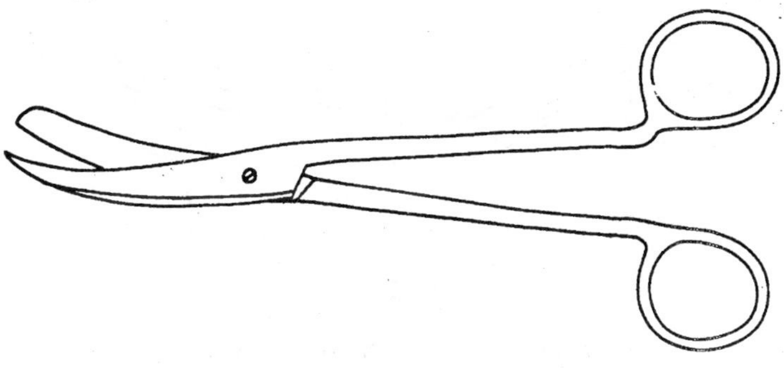

Figure 8.10 : Curved on flat scissors

3. Curved on angle scissors.

(a) Heath ligature scissors: It is a curved on angle type of scissors. The curvature at the tip is in the same horizontal plane. One of the blades has serrations to hook the stitches which are cut after steadving them with a toothed forceps.

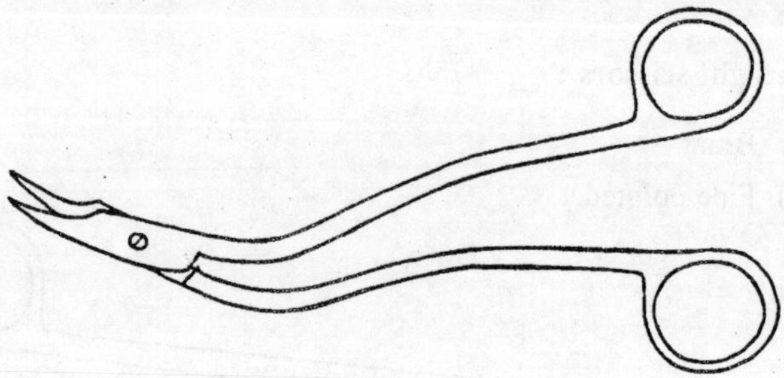

Figure 8.11 : Heath ligature scissors

(b) Episiotomy scissors: This is a curved on angle type of scissors with blunt tips so that it can not damage any structure. One blade has lateral serrations for a secure grip of the tissue to give a smooth and straight incision without ragged edges.

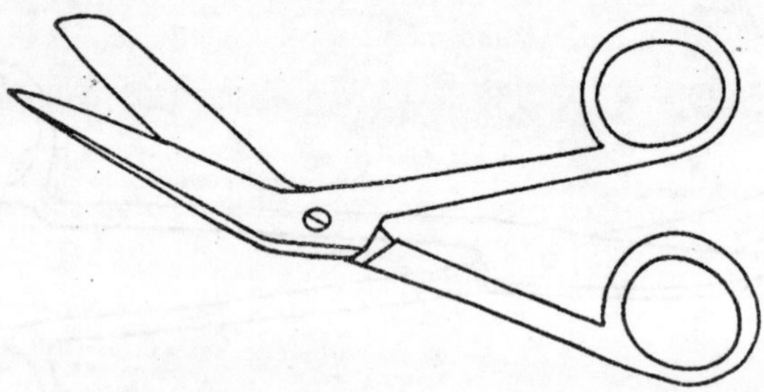

Figure 8.12 : Episiotomy scissors

Uses

1. For blunt dissection in tissues containing lots of connective tissue. The scissors may be used here with closed blades which are opened up in various directions to break the connective tissue.
2. For sharp dissection, etc. to push down an adherent bladder from the lower uterine segment in a case of previous LSCS. The tips are used here to cut the adhesions.

3. Can be used for extending a skin incision in place of scalpel and for cutting pedicles and sutures.

BARD PARKER'S KNIFE HANDLE WITH BLADE

It is a simple, straight handle with a notch where different disposable blades can be attached according to the requirement of the surgeon.

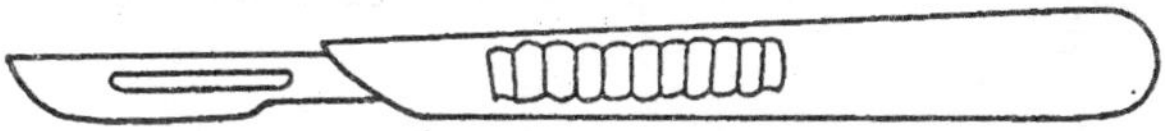

Figure 8.13: Bard Parker's knife handle with blade

Uses

1. For opening the abdomen.
2. For sharp dissection.
3. For cutting pedicles.

RAMPLEY'S SPONGE HOLDING FORCEPS

It is a long forceps with 2 blades, a handle with finger grips and a lock. The blades are ring like, fenestrated and have transverse serrations. The transverse serrations on blades and the lock provide a firm grip but cause minimal trauma as the blades are rounded and blunt.

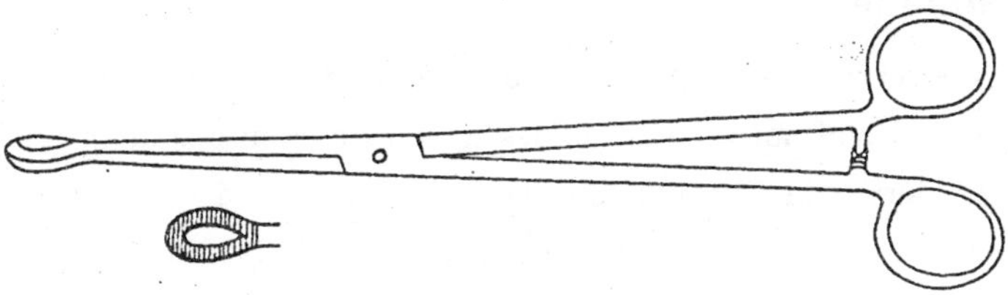

Figure 8.14 : Rampley's sponge holding forceps

Uses

1. For cleaning and dressing of the patient.
2. For swabbing a cavity, e.g. the uterus in lower segment caesarean section and vaginal wash down.
3. The transverse serrations help in making the instrument a good haemostat so can be used for holding the angles in caesarean section.
4. For packing a cavity, e.g. vagina in cervical tears.
5. For holding small rounded pieces of gauze for mopping the operative field.
6. Holding the cervix in pregnancy when the cervix is soft and the toothed volsellum can injure it, e.g. for MacDonald's stitches.
7. In place of an ovum forceps in PPH, incomplete abortion and septic abortion.
8. For holding the terminal part of membranes while delivering placenta.
9. May be used as a clamp, e.g. clamping of umblical cord, etc.

ABDOMINAL RETRACTORS

These are used to obtain a good exposure of the operative field for performing better surgery. They help the surgeon by enlarging the operative field, preventing damage to the adjacent structures, prevent undue handling of tissues and save time. The bleeding areas are better exposed and bleeders are more easily caught and tied.

Technique

The retractor should always be introduced along the long axis of the wound and not at right angles to it to minimise trauma to the wound during its introduction. The traction should be gentle and tissues should not be put under undue tension. If greater force is required and the surgeon apprehends damage to the tissues then a linen pack should be inserted in between the tissue and the retractor.

Type of Retractors : They can be of two types.

(i) Plain retractors which are non-self retaining.

(ii) Self retaining retractors

I. PLAIN RETRACTORS

These are simple in design consisting of a blade for retraction a shaft and a handle for holding the retractor from a distance with a good grip. The advantage with plain retractors is that they can be moved and manipulated as and when required in a convenient and simple manner. The following are some examples of plain retractors.

CZERNY'S RETRACTOR

It is a plain, non-self retaining retractor consisting of a small blade at one end, a shaft and a biflanged hook on the other end. The two ends are directed in opposite directions. The shaft is fenestrated to make the instrument light.

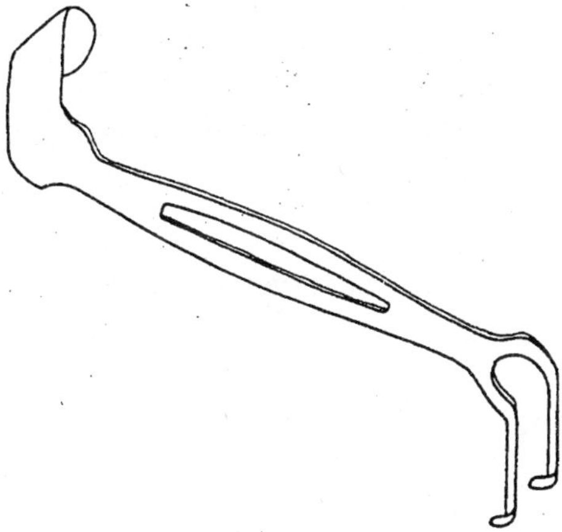

Figure 8.15 : Czerny's retractor

Uses

1. It is used to retract abdominal incisions.
2. The biflanged end may be used to take the last deep stitch during wound closure.

DOYEN'S RETRACTOR

It is a strong, heavy non-self retaining abdominal retractor. It consists of a large blade which is curved having an inward turning margins to minimise trauma to the abdominal wall during retraction. The retractor comes in different sizes. It can be converted to a self retaining type by hanging lead weights from the hook present on the handle.

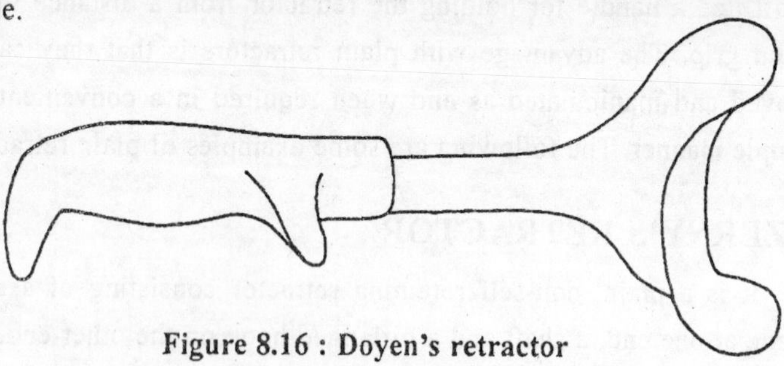

Figure 8.16 : Doyen's retractor

Uses

1. In all abdominal surgery.
2. Specially useful for deep pelvic surgery.

DELEE'S UNIVERSAL RETRACTOR

This instrument is similar to a Doyen's retractor except that the curve of the blade here is of greater depth and the instrument is lighter because of presence of fenestrated handles which also help in providing a better grip.

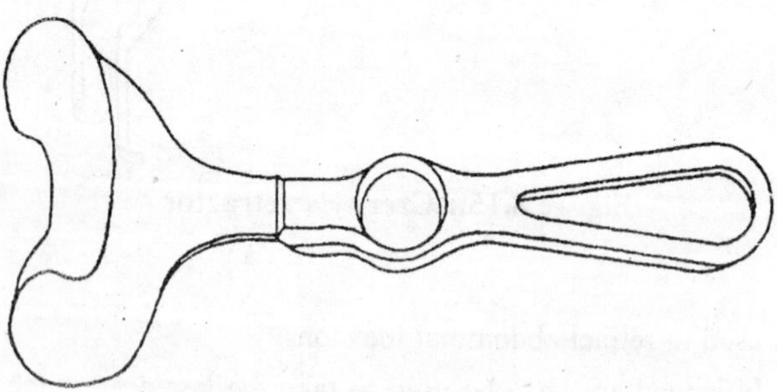

Figure 8.17 : Delee's universal retractor

Uses

1. In all abdominal operations.
2. In all operations in the pelvis.

MIKULICZ'S RETRACTOR

It consists of a long and thin strip of metal forming the blade of the retractor. It has fenestrated stout handle. The retractor occupies little space as it is thin and is used to retract upper abdominal structures, e.g. liver, etc. The retractor may be covered by a linen pad to prevent damage to the underlying structure. The length and curvature make it ideal for retraction when operating in depth but as it is a light instrument it cannot effectively retract the thick abdominal wall.

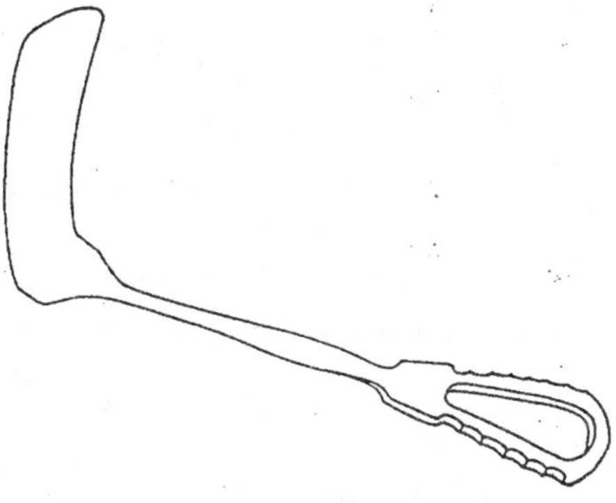

Figure 8.18 : Mikulicz's retractor

Uses

During abdominal operations, like internal iliac ligation, sling operations, etc. to retract the intra-peritoneal structures.

II. SELF RETAINING ABDOMINAL RETRACTOR

The instrument consists of movable blades the position of which can be fixed by screw locks. The advantage of this type of retractor is that the assistant is free to participate actively in surgery. Also, correct and uniform amount of traction is possible throughout the operation.

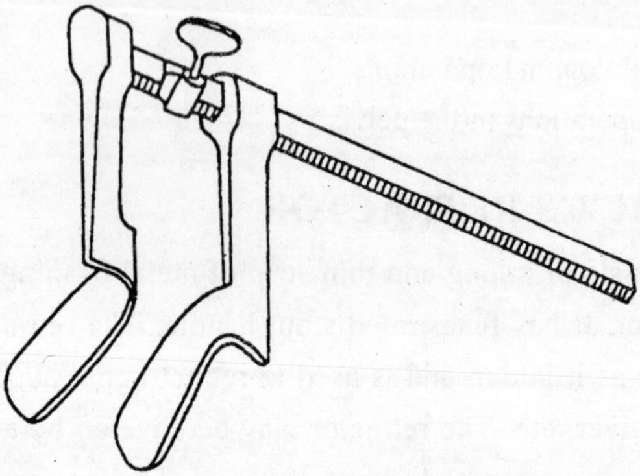

Figure 8.19 : Self retaining abdominal retractor

Uses

1. It is used in operations where prolonged surgery is planned.
2. Where the surgery is difficult and more active participation of assistants is needed it is of great help

CATHETERS AND DRAINS

These are long tubular structures of plastic, rubber or metal used for draining fluids from body cavities.

PLAIN OR SIMPLE RUBBER CATHETER

It is a simple non self retaining red coloured rubber tube having a blunt end with an opening subterminally for drainage. The other end is slightly expanded. It comes in various sizes depending on the diameter of the tube.

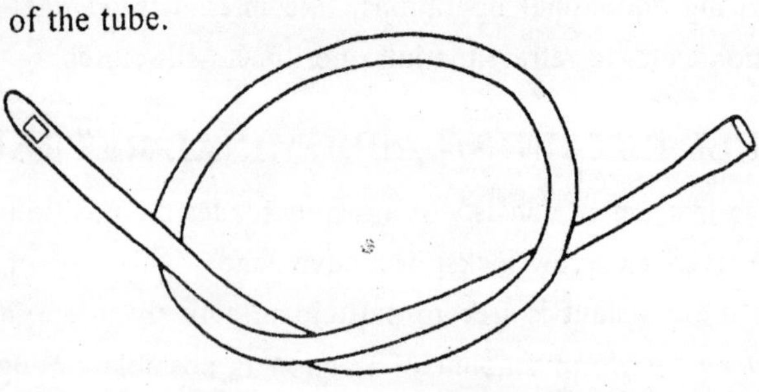

Figure 8.20 : Simple rubber catheter

Uses

It is used for a single urethral catheterization as its prolonged stay in the urethra can lead to certain harmful chemical changes in the rubber tubing.

K-90 NELATON'S SIMPLE CATHETER

This is a plastic type, non self-retaining catheter with a blunt tip and a subterminal opening. The plastic is rigid polyvinyl hence it is easier to pass specially in obstetrical patients when the descent of the fetal head prevents easy catheterisation.

Use

For a single urethral catheterisation.

FOLEY'S SELF RETAINING CATHETER

It is a soft rubber catheter which may be 2 or 3 channelled. The tip has a subterminal hole for drainage and beyond this lies a balloon which can be inflated to make the catheter self-retaining. The capacity of the balloon varies between 5-50 cc and is mentioned on the package. The main channel is for drainage, another one is for inflating the balloon while a third channel may be present which can be used for irrigation of the bladder.

During catheterisation there may be a problem in insertion as it is a soft rubber catheter when a rigid metallic tube may be used known as catheter inserter. The catheter is available in various sizes according to the French scale where:

$$\text{Diameter of catheter in mm} = \frac{\text{Catheter number}}{3}$$

Thus diameter of the catheter increases with the increase in number. The usual size for an adult female is No. 14 or No. 16.

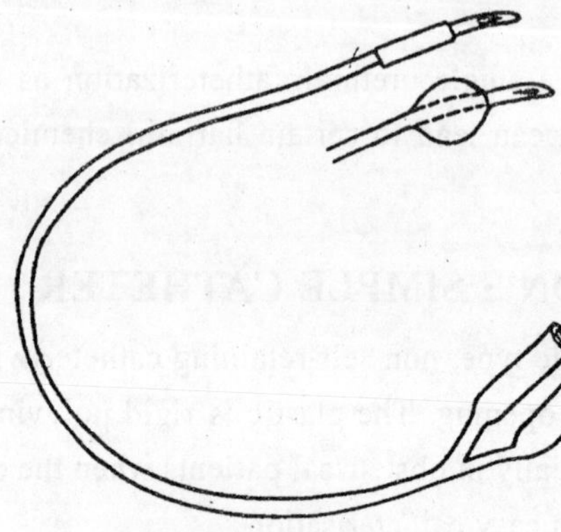

Figure 8.21 : Foley's catheter

Technique

The catheterisation of the patient should be done only if clearly indicated. A no-touch aseptic technique should be used. The patient is put in the lithotomy position, the vulva and perineum are cleaned and labia are retracted away to clean the urethra from above downwards and not in the opposite direction. The labia should not be allowed to fall back. The correct size of the catheter is chosen. The urethral meatus is the narrowest part of the urethra and the size of the catheter is decided by the size of the meatus. The catheter is inserted keeping the inner covering intact and only tip of the catheter is exposed. The normal length of the female urethra is 3–4 cm and this much of the catheter should go in beyond the balloon. This is important as otherwise the balloon may be inflated in the urethra, damaging it. Pushing in more length of the catheter than this is unnecessary as it increases chances of infection. The balloon is inflated with normal saline and the urethral dressing is done by rolling sterile gauze all round the catheter near the meatus. The catheter is then taped to one side of the patient's thigh such that the level remains below the level of the urethra. The catheter tubing should also be fixed to the bed clothes to prevent kinking and then joined to a closed drainage system, a urobag. The catheter is removed by simply puncturing the same channel which was used for inflating by a needle and removing the fluid. Sometimes it becomes difficult to deflate the balloon. Ether can be pushed in which causes the balloon to burst. Alternatively the balloon can be palpated per vaginum and punctured with a needle from the vagina. In prolonged catheterisations the catheter should be removed after intermittent clamping to retrain the bladder otherwise it may result in the retention of urine due to loss of bladder tone.

Indications of Catheterisation

1. Acute retention of urine not relieved by conservative methods.
2. Chronic retention of urine, in this case slow decompression should be done.
3. Neurogenic bladder.
4. Surgery on the bladder, e.g. VVF repair, bladder rupture, etc.
5. All pelvic operations, e.g. vaginal hysterectomy, abdominal hysterectomy so that the field is not obstructed by a full bladder and to avoid reflex retention in post operative period.
6. In vaginal operations to prevent accidental damage.
7. In obstructed labour to prevent formation of a vesicovaginal fistula.
8. For instillation of antiseptic, chemotherapeutic and diagnostic agents into the bladder.
9. To measure residual urine, bladder capacity, etc.
10. For cystourethrography
11. For assessment of the total urine output in acute renal failure, chronic renal failure, congestive cardiac failure and other medical diseases.
12. In unconscious patients to prevent soiling of clothes.
13. In antepartum hemorrhage, post partum hemorrhage to control bleeding.
14. During labour when the patient is unable to void urine and prior to delivery by forceps or ventouse.

15. For hysterosalpingography, hydrotubation of fallopian tubes, emcredil insertion and after drainage of pyometra or haematometra the catheter may be inserted in the uterus through the cervical canal.
16. Drainage of any other body cavity.
17. To identify the bladder neck in Kelly's repair operation.

Complications

1. Acute urinary tract infection.
2. Chronic urinary tract infection.
3. Prolonged catheterisation may result in loss of bladder tone.

MALECOT'S CATHETER

It is a self retaining catheter used for draining body cavities. It has a bulbous winged tip. The catheter is introduced after straightening the bulbous tip by stretching it over an artery clamp. When the forceps is removed the elastic recoil of the catheter re-forms the tip into bulbous form and it becomes a self-retaining type of catheter. The advantage is that it can be easily removed by gentle pulling. It comes in various sizes, the diameter being directly proportional to the number of the catheter. The large sized catheters are used for draining thick secretions like pus and blood, etc. while the small sized are used for thinner serous or sero-sanguinous secretions whenever drainage of a cavity is required.

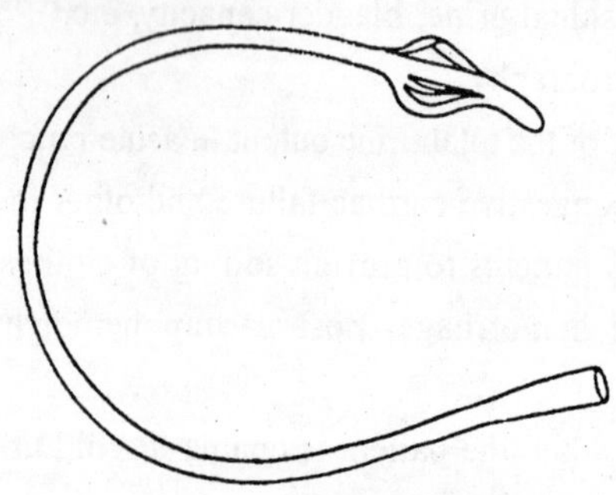

Figure 8.22 : Malecot's catheter

SUTURE MATERIALS

For quick healing of a wound the essential requirements are well apposed edges with meticulous hemostasis. Suture materials are threaded on needles and used for passing ligatures for approximation and homeostasis. Selection of an appropriate suture material is of immense importance for a strong and cosmetically pleasing scar. Two main types of suture materials are used:

1. Absorbable :

(a) Plain catgut
(b) Chromic catgut
(c) Polygalactin 910 or Vicryl
(d) Polyglycolic acid or Dexon, etc.

2. Non absorbable :

(a) Nylon
(b) Cotton
(c) Silk
(d) Steel
(e) Prolene, etc.

Sutures are divided into different sizes based on their diameter. Sutures progressively larger than no. 0 are numbered in increasing numeric order (no. 1, 2 etc.) sizes progressively smaller than 0–0 are indicated by an increasing number of zeros (e.g. 0,00, 000). The smaller the suture diameter, the more the zeros. For simplicity the smaller numbers are often written 1–0, 2–0 with the first numeral referring to the number of zeros.

Choice of a suture material

The right suture materials to use in a particular situation depends on the following factors:

1. Whether the suture is absorbable or non-absorbable:

Absorbable sutures are digested by the enzyme systems or

by phagocytosis while non-absorbable ones are unaffected by biological activities and are permanent unless removed. They become encapsulated by fibrous tissue after sometime. Thus slow healing tissues like fascia and skin may be sutured by nonabsorbable sutures while rapidly healing tissues like stomach, peritoneum, vagina can be repaired by absorbable or non-absorbable both.

2. Tensile strength of the sutures :

It is the minimum amount of tension or weight required to break the suture. Non absorbable sutures have a greater tensile strength.

3. Tissue reaction elicited by the sutures :

Absorbable sutures elicit a stronger tissue reaction with more chances of sepsis while non-absorbable ones are less irritant and promote quicker healing with a stronger wound.

4. Filament arrangement of the material :

The suture may be monofilament type or polyfilament type which may be twisted or braided. The polyfilaments have higher tensile strength with stronger knots but the roughened surface has more chances of inviting sepsis. The monofilament is smooth with lesser chances of infection but tensile strength is less and knots tend to slip. Some polyfilament sutures are chemically treated to smoothen the surface so that chances of infection are reduced.

5. Ease of sterilisation :

An ideal suture material is one which can be easily sterilised without decreasing its tensile strength or changing its physico-chemical properties.

6. Presence of infection:

Here monofilament absorbable sutures are better but stronger ones should be used because of increased breakdown of the sutures in presence of infection and delayed healing so monofilament delayed absorbable sutures should be used.

7. Cosmetic results :

Inert non-absorbable fine sutures should be used for better cosmetic results.

8. Undernourished, anaemic and hypoproteinemic patients:

Here healing is delayed so the wound has to be kept approximated for a longer time. Non-absorbable or delayed absorbable sutures should be preferred.

9. Collagen content of tissue :

Tissues with a high amount of collagen, e.g., fascia, tendon, aponeurosis, etc. require a longer time to heal and so non-absorbable or delayed absorbable sutures should be used:

I. ABSORBABLE SUTURES

Surgical catgut :

It is an absorbable suture material known to surgeons since the time of Galen (AD 131-210). It is manufactured from collagen derived from the intestinal mucosa of cow or sheep which has a high tensile strength due to the presence of lots of elastic tissue. Lord Lister (1827-1912) played an important role in its development. He treated it with 20% chromic acid making it more inert with lesser tissue reaction as it binds to the antigen sites of the collagen. Thus the chromic catgut has more tensile strength, delayed absorption with lesser amount of tissue reaction. It is available in dark tan to yellowish brown colour ranging in size from No. 7–0 to 3. and a length of 5 feet. Three knots should be applied for safety as catgut swells up before being dissolved. It loses 70% of tensile strength by 7 days and is totally absorbed in 70 days.

Uses are for suturing rapidly healing tissues like mucosa, peritoneum, etc. Disadvantage is the variability of absorption. In presence of infection the tensile strength decreases rapidly as degradation by proteases released by white blood cells is increased.

Vicryl or Polyglactin 910 :

It is a synthetic suture available in sizes varying from 9–0 to 3. It is a polyfilament, braided suture which is dyed violet for easy recognition. The loss in tensile strength is 40% by 2nd week and 70% by the 3rd week. The absorption is minimal by 40th day and then is rapidly absorbed between 60–90 days. The absorption is by slow hydrolysis in tissue fluids. Four knots should be tied for safety. Tissue reaction is less, tensile strength and absorption are not affected in presence of infection as the absorption is by hydrolysis and it does not undergo enzymatic degradation. It is used where prolonged approximation of tissues is required and slow healing is expected. The disadvantage is that as the suture is polyfilament braided it causes tissue drag and infection spreads fast due to the irregular surface.

Dexon or Polyglycolic acid suture :

It is a synthetic delayed absorbable braided suture. The filaments are dyed green to enhance visibility in tissues. The size varies from 8–0 to 2. The suture looses 40–50% of its tensile strength by 2 weeks and 80% by 3 weeks. Tissue reaction is minimal and fine fibrous connective tissue grows into and over the suture increasing tensile strength of the wound. Absorption starts within 2 weeks and is over in 60–90 days but is slower than that of vicryl and unaffected in presence of infection. The suture is chemically treated to make its surface smooth to prevent infection but the disadvantage is that knot security is poor and at least 6 knots are needed for safety. It is used for subcutaneous fascial and peritoneal repair specially for infected wounds as degradation product is bactericidal and the smoothened surface prevents spread of infection.

Polyglyconate and Polydioxanane (PDS)

It is a pliable monofilament, synthetic, delayed absorbable suture. Initial tensile strength is high but absorption is much delayed so tensile strength is maintained for much longer and 25% of it remains by 6 weeks. Inflammatory response is minimal as is monofilament also spread of infection is less.

II. NON ABSORBABLE SUTURES

Nylon or Polyamide polymer :

It is a synthetic monofilament polyamide polymer. It is available in sizes ranging from 11–0 to 2. It is dyed green or black and is chemically treated to make its surface smooth and non-capillary in action. It is less irritant and stronger than surgical silk. The degradation per year is by 15–20% and there occurs a gradual loss in its tensile strength. It causes minimal tissue reaction, with no drag on the tissues while pulling, is elastic in nature and of good tensile strength. The knots however tend to slip and atleast 6–7 knots are needed. It is used for skin closure for subcuticular stitches, as retention suture for herniorrhaphy, for tendon repair and as pull out sutures.

Prolene or polypropylene :

It is a synthetic polymer having indefinite in-vivo tensile strength. It is monofilament, non-capillary and is dyed blue. The sizes available range from 10–0 to 1. It is almost inert and elicits minimal tissue reaction. It is unaffected by tissue fluids and can be used in the presence of infection. At least 5–6 knots should be applied. It is used for general closure, vascular surgery, tuboplasty and as a pull out suture.

Surgical Silk :

It is a protein thread secreted by the silkworm for its cocoon. The fibres are processed to remove their natural waxes and gums and twisted or braided to form strands. Though grouped under non-absorbable, it looses most of its tensile strength by 1 year and is absorbed by the second year. It is dyed black to improve visibility in tissues and is chemically treated to remove its capillary action. The suture is available in sizes from 9–0 to 5. The tensile strength decreases in presence of moisture so it is used dry. It has a moderate tensile strength and elicits moderate tissue reaction. The advantage is easy handling with a secure knot. The disadvantage is low tensile strength and tendency to serve as a nidus in presence of infection.

Surgical Cotton :

It is made from cotton fibres which are straightened, aligned and twisted into strands. The tensile strength is low and 50% is lost by 6 months and 80% by 2 years. The suture frays easily. The sizes available range from 3–0 to 2. The tissue response is minimal for each strand but once braided together they elicit a strong reaction and should not be used in infected tissues. The tensile strength increases when wet but handling becomes difficult. It has no advantage over silk except its lower cost.

Chapter IX

Endoscopy in Obstetrics and Gynaecology

Endoscopy is the visualisation of body cavities by specialised instruments or endoscopes. Endoscopes are now being used with increasing frequency both for diagnostic and therapeutic indications. The various types used in obstetrics and gynaecology are laparoscope, amnioscope; hysteroscope; salpingoscope; culdoscope, fetoscope, etc.

Laparoscopy is the visualisation of abdominal cavity for therapeutic and diagnostic purposes. A brief discussion of the instruments required, technique and complications is given below.

Insufflation Needle

The veress needle is the most commonly used insufflation needle for producing a pneumo-peritoneum. It is a long needle 4-6 inches in length and has a spring mechanism. The needle consists of an outer sheath having a sharp edge and an inner blunt stylet which protrudes beyond the sharp edge for half a centimeter. When the needle is pushed through the tougher structures of the sheath the spring mechanism allows the blunt inner needle to be pushed up and the sharp end protrude out which allows easy penetration. When the needle reaches the peritoneum and other soft structures inside the abdominal cavity the blunt inner needle protrudes out as the upward thrust on the spring mechanism is released. The needle has a connection for the CO_2 source and allows a flow rate of 1 litre/minute.

CO_2 insufflator

It is used to produce a controlled pneumo-peritoneum. It is a separate unit with dials indicating the volume of CO_2 in the peritoneal cavity and the rate of flow of the gas. The use of CO_2 for pneumoperitoneum has the highest degree of safety as it diffuses rapidly due to its high solubility. It causes least pain and danger of embolism is less as compared to air or nitrous oxide. The newer fully automated CO_2 insufflators deliver gas under optimal pressure by automatic increase or decrease in the rate of flow and thus maintain the optimal intra-abdominal pressure required by the surgeon. Systems which deliver preheated gas at 37°C are also available. The advantage here is that there is no danger of the patient going into shock because of exposure to cold gas. The rate of flow of gas should be around 10–15 liters/minute but a rate as high as 30 liters/minute may be needed for laser surgery.

Trocars and Canulae

These come in various sizes and are used as portals for introducing various instruments into the abdominal cavity. A sharp penetrating trocar 1–1.5 cm in diameter protrudes out of an outer blunt canula. The trocar may be conical or pyramidal at the tip. The canula may have a trumpet or flapper valve which allows entry of instruments but prevents leakage of gas. The canula has a channel for connecting with the gas delivery system. Trocars have the tendency to slip out during prolonged surgery so cannulae having spiral or grooved outer surfaces which prevent slipping may be used.

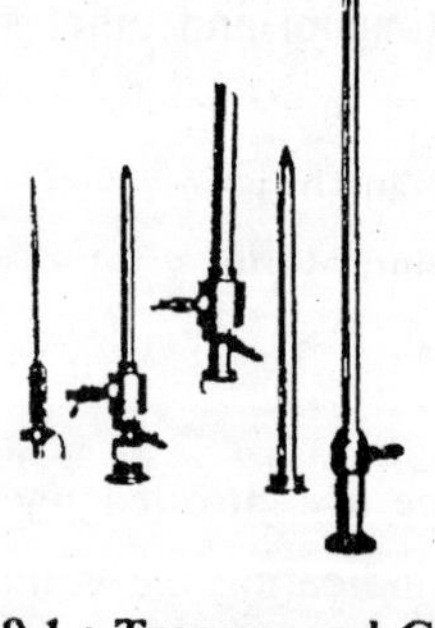

Figure 9.1 : Trocars and Canulae

Laparoscope

It consists of a telescope with an objective and an eye piece and a light conducting system. The presently used operative telescopes have large diameters (10–12 mm) and have an additional channel for introduction of operative instruments. The light is transmitted by a fiber-optic bundle from a light source having a fan for dissipation of heat and hence it is also known as a 'cold light source'. This fiber-optic light conducting system has more than 2 million fibres. The angle of vision of a laparoscope may be either 'zero degrees' or 'thirty degree fore oblique' and the viewer must get adapted to this viewing angle. The eyepiece may be either perpendicular, angled or oblique, or it may be parallel type. The number of prisms is reduced in perpendicular or oblique type and therefore there is more clarity and brightness of image. The magnification achieved is a product of the linear magnification of the objective and visual magnification of the eyepiece. At an object distance of 5 cm the magnification is one, i.e., an object viewed from a 5 cm distance will be seen in its actual size. The laparoscope is sterilised by exposure to formalin vapours or immersion in glutaraldehyde and cleared with normal saline before use.

Anaesthesia

Though diagnostic laparoscopy and minor surgical procedures lasting for 5-10 minutes may be done under sedation prolonged laparoscopic surgery requires a relaxed abdominal wall for better visualisation. Light anaesthesia allowing activity of abdominal muscles can increase the intra abdominal pressure and thus stop the inflow of gas from the automatic insufflator preventing the proper visualisation of structures. It must be remembered that the anaesthetic agents used should not be inflammable. The trendelenberg position of the patient and the use of CO_2 for pneumoperitoneum increases the chances of acidosis so there should be controlled ventilation and the end tidal

CO_2 volume monitoring should be done throughout the surgery. There is also a danger of injury to bowel and other structures if the patient is light and pushes the intestines. Thus good general anaesthesia, administered by an experienced and trained anaesthetist is an essential requirement for laparoscopic surgery.

Light Source

The quality of endoscopic surgery depends on adequate visualisation. This in turn depends on the quality and power of the light delivered to the laparoscope which is the net result of the lamps, cables, etc. The light sources available are Halogen (150–250 w), Halide (250–400 w) and Xenon (175 & 300 w). The Xenon is the most powerful light source but it is also the most expensive. Halogen lamps are the cheapest. The light source delivers this cold light via fiber-optic light cables varying from 3.5–6.0 mm in diameter. Larger diameter cables give better intensity light. Fluid cables which transmit light via fluid medium are also available and in these advantage is that they do not wear out with time.

Video Camera and Monitors

The advantages of using a video system during laparoscopic surgery are :

(a) The surgeon can operate for a long period without bending his back.

(b) The assistants can help more actively during surgery.

(c) The beginners have an opportunity for observing and learning.

(d) The procedure can be recorded and the tapes can be replayed if any complications occur in the post operative period.

The highly advanced CCD or 'charge – coupled – device camera' gives images of high quality and is very small and light weight. The camera may have a single silicon chip or may be 3–chip type with a very high resolution power. The camera has to be 'white balanced' before use by directing it towards a pure white background so that it gives an accurate spectrum of colours. There is usually an automatic focussing device and a manual device for adjusting the light intensity. Zooming in facility is also available in some cameras but these are very expensive.

Monitors are used one on each side of the patient for the comfort of the surgeon and his assistants. The screen should be at least 13 inches for adequate visibility.

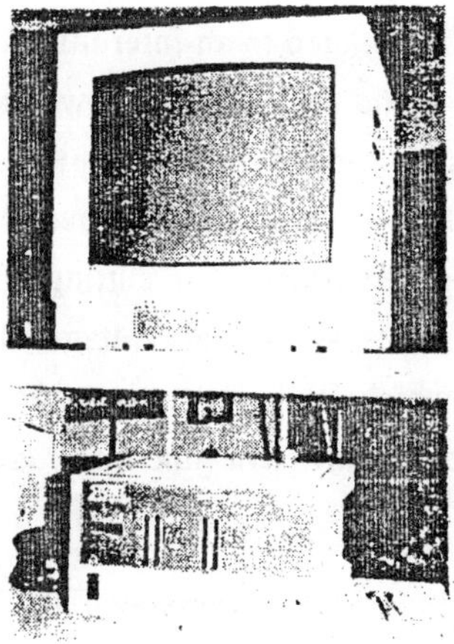

Figure 9.2 : Video monitor and insufflator

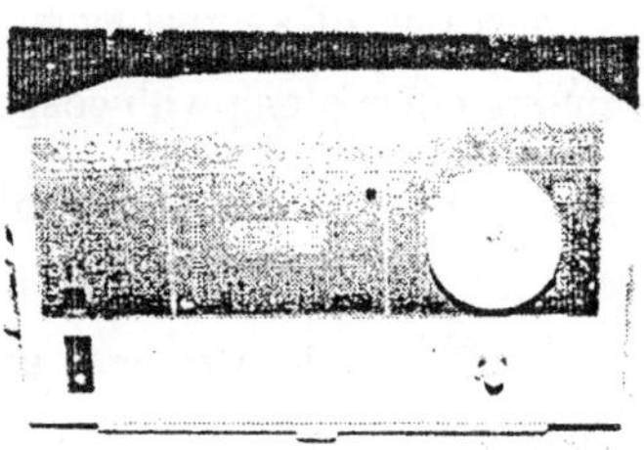

Figure 9.3 : Light source

Electrosurgical Unit

They are used for cutting or coagulating human tissue depending on the nature of the current used. The thermal effect of high frequency electric current is utilised for this. The thickness and shape of the electrode decides the effect of the current, e.g.:

(a) Thin edged needle/knife electrode will perform the function of cutting.

(b) A thick needle or a ball electrodes will perform coagulation with the same voltage.

The current is modulated to an intermittent flow so that the heating of tissues is slow and the tissue is allowed to cool in between and to prevent local tissue vaporisation. The higher the voltage used the longer the modulation interval required and the greater coagulation effect for achieving hemostasis. For cutting effect it is necessary to have a high continuous sinusoidal voltage. This generates a high local temperature which leads to cutting effect but as the tissue is heated swiftly there is insufficient time for coagulation and hemostasis here is less.

There are three types of currents available.

1. Continuous sinusoidal cutting current (low voltage, high frequency)
2. Modulated coagulation current (high voltage, low frequency)
3. Blended waveform current which is a combination of cutting and coagulation types consisting of alternating high and low voltage. This produces a cutting effect along with coagulation.

A good cautery machine which can deliver all the three types of current at varying voltages for use in various situations and at the same time one which is able to deliver both unipolar and bipolar current should be available to the surgeon.

In unipolar current the electrons seek a pathway to ground and there is a risk of injury if an organ is accidently touched. In bipolar current, to burn a structure the operator must grasp the tissue in between the prongs of the forceps, i.e., the bipolar design limits the current to the two prongs of the grasping forceps and the tissue held in between. Therefore chances of accidental injuries is less in this case.

Suction Irrigation Unit

This consists of a delivery system which pushes an irrigating fluid under force, e.g. Ringer's lactate or Normal saline through a canula 4–10 mm in diameter.

This wide bore canula can remove blood clots and tissue pieces from the peritoneal cavity but disadvantage is that it can also suck out a large amount of gas so a small bore canula is preferred. This can also be used for hydro-dissection, e.g. separating the two layers of the broad ligament. They can deliver fluid at the rate of 1500 ml/minute. Blunt and needle tipped aspirators are available for aspiration of ovarian cysts, fluid in cul-de-sac, etc. These can be used manually or attached to suction devices.

Operating Instruments

The various instruments required are :

(a) grasping forceps which may be toothed or non toothed and may have a sharp or a rounded tip;
(b) scissors which may be straight curved or hooked;
(c) needle holders;
(d) clips, staples, etc.

Technique

The procedure may be done under IV sedation or general anaesthesia depending upon its duration. The position of the patient is trendelenberg with lower limbs fixed to low stirrups as in lithotomy position. Pneumoperitoneum is created with the help of the veress needle and this helps by pushing away the bowel loops and omentum and also helps by tenting the abdominal wall. The veress needle with stylet is introduced through a stab incision below the umbilicus. The needle should enter at an angle of 90° and its entry is confirmed by pushing in 20 ml of saline. If inside the peritoneal cavity the saline can not be aspirated back (Palmer's test). It is now connected to the CO_2 insufflator. The stab incision is now enlarged and the trocar and canula are introduced by gentle screwing movements again at an angle of 45° to the abdominal wall. Once the peritoneum is pierced the trocar is pulled up while the canula is pushed in so that viscera may not be damaged by the sharp tip of the trocar. The laparoscope is now introduced through the canula and the peritoneal cavity can be visualised for diagnostic and operative procedures.

Complications of Laparoscopic Surgery

1. Bowel injury by trocar or veress needle
2. Vascular injuries.
3. Injury to the bladder or ureters.
4. Cardiac arrest or arrhythmias.
5. Anaesthetic complications.
6. Haemorrhage.
7. Omental prolapse through puncture site.
8. Sepsis.
9. Embolism.
10. Surgical emphysema.

Index